RENEWALS 458-4574

DATE DUE

GAYLORD | | | PRINTED IN U.S.A.

Self-Trust and Reproductive Autonomy

Basic Bioethics
Glenn McGee and Arthur Caplan, series editors

Self-Trust and Reproductive Autonomy

Carolyn McLeod

A Bradford Book

The MIT Press
Cambridge, Massachusetts
London, England

This book was set in Sabon by Northeastern Graphic Services, Inc.
Printed and bound in the United States of America.

Library of Congress Cataloging-in-Publication Data
McLeod, Carolyn.
  Self-trust and reproductive autonomy / Carolyn McLeod.
  p. cm.—(Basic bioethics)
  Includes bibliographic references and index.
  ISBN 0-262-13408-X (hc. : alk. paper)
  1. Human reproductive technology—Moral and ethical aspects.
2. Human reproduction—Moral and ethical aspects. 3. Autonomy.
4. Medical ethics. 5. Bioethics. 6. Trust. 7. Feminism—Health aspects.
8. Feminism—Moral and ethical aspects. 9. Ethics I. Title. II. Series.

RG133.5 .M39   2002
176—dc21   2001055809

For my parents,
Mary Anne and Rod McLeod,
and my siblings,
Andy and Katie McLeod

Contents

Series Foreword

We are pleased to present the fifth volume in the series Basic Bioethics. The series presents innovative book-length manuscripts in bioethics to a broad audience and introduces seminal scholarly manuscripts, state-of-the-art reference works, and textbooks. Such broad areas as the philosophy of medicine, advancing genetics and biotechnology, end of life care, health and social policy, and the empirical study of biomedical life will be engaged.

Glenn McGee
Arthur Caplan

Acknowledgments

Many people nurtured the self-trust that allowed me to complete this project. Foremost among them are Susan Sherwin and Richmond Campbell. Sue was extremely generous with her time and gave me pointed and insightful criticism at early stages of writing. I am indebted to her for challenging me in an insistent yet supportive way. Rich provided excellent philosophical advice as well as sympathy whenever I lost self-trust, particularly at a crucial stage in chapter 6. He and Sue inspire me with their commitment to feminist philosophy and to the development of young scholars.

Sue Campbell and Duncan McIntosh read numerous drafts and gave extensive comments. I benefited from Sue's mastery of feminist moral psychology and her finely tuned perception of its relevance to women's lives. I was fortunate early on to have Duncan nearby while he was on sabbatical, and on more occasions than I remember, I mined his philosophical knowledge and relied on his enhanced decision-making skills.

I am also grateful to Diana Meyers for reading the manuscript and giving me detailed suggestions, all of which I tried to incorporate into the final version. Her work has hugely shaped my understanding of autonomy and of the barriers posed to it by sexism. I owe an intellectual debt also to Annette Baier, whose insights on trust are profound, in my view, and whose style and wit made researching the subject a joy.

It was rewarding for me to challenge philosophical assumptions about trust, autonomy, and reproductive freedom against the background of women's reproductive lives. I thank the women whose stories I used for their honesty and willingness to contribute to the literature on women's reproductive health. I especially thank Lee Harris and the women who consented to having me observe their prenatal visits as part of a clinical practicum I did in obstetrics. Françoise Baylis and Barbara Parish organized and supervised that experience. They introduced me, respectively, to the complicated yet fascinating worlds of clinical bioethics and modern obstetrical care, and for that, I am grateful.

Carolyn Gray Anderson was a pleasure to work with at the MIT Press, and I am glad that we had a chance to meet in London at the conference of Feminist Approaches to Bioethics. She solicited many reviews from competent academics, including Susan Dodds, who agreed to review the manuscript twice. I truly appreciated her interest in the project and her comments on drafts.

Parts of the manuscript have been presented or published elsewhere. An earlier version of my philosophical views on self-trust and autonomy exists in a piece I coauthored with Sue Sherwin called "Relational Autonomy, Self-Trust, and Health Care for Patients Who are Oppressed" (in *Relational Autonomy: Feminist Perspectives on Autonomy, Agency, and the Social Self,* edited by Catriona Mackenzie and Natalie Stoljar). I appreciated having the opportunity to develop those ideas in print. Much of chapter 2 appears as "Our Attitude Towards the Motivation of Those We Trust" (2000) in *The Southern Journal of Philosophy,* vol. 38, no. 3: 465–479 (reprinted with permission). I also gave drafts of different chapters at conferences held by the Canadian Society for Women in Philosophy, the Canadian Philosophical Association, and the Canadian Bioethics Society, and at the philosophy departments at the University of Calgary, McGill University, York University, the University of Tennessee (Knoxville), and Dalhousie University. I received some crucial feedback at those events, and I heartily thank my audiences.

Work on this project (and others) has taken me to three different cities in the past three years. I revised the manuscript while on a two-year Social Sciences and Humanities Research Council (SSHRC) of Canada postdoctoral fellowship. The first year I spent at the Bioethics Center at the University of Minnesota, where I was offered a second fellowship. Carl Elliott supervised my work and gave me invaluable advice, particularly on reworking chapter 3.

For the second year of my SSHRC fellowship, I went to the philosophy department at the University of Western Ontario to work with Samantha Brennan on feminist ethics. Samantha read the entire manuscript and gave me encouraging feedback. Along with Tracy Isaacs, Kathleen Okruhlik, and other feminist faculty, she welcomed me wholeheartedly into a stimulating community of feminist academics. Dennis Klimchuk also was an excellent colleague as well as my neighbor for that year. He spurred me on with his enthusiasm upon reading parts of the manuscript, and he provided some tasty meals and good company for Walter, Lenny, and me.

The final touches were made at the University of Tennessee, Knoxville. I have gladly become immersed in a vibrant and friendly department that is committed to research and teaching, along with practical methods of pursuing philosophy.

Among those who gave me support and kept me smiling (most of the time) throughout my many moves are Sian Owen, Colleen Flood, David McCallum, Vaughan Black, Christine Koggel, Ariella Pahlke, Phlis McGregor, and John Lougheed. I am grateful for their e-mails, their long-distance calls, and the precious time I have been able to spend with them in the past few years.

Last, it gives me immense pleasure to dedicate this book to my parents, who have provided me with a firm foundation of love and respect that I carry with me everywhere. I also dedicate the book to my brother and sister, who have filled my life with support, laughter, and a little healthy competition. In ways they hardly realize, my whole family, including my sister-in-law Shelagh, are largely responsible for the self-trust that fuels my commitment to feminist academics and to justice in reproductive health care for women.

Self-Trust and Reproductive Autonomy

1

Introduction: Minimizing Patient Vulnerability by Valuing Self-Trust

Because of increasing medicalization of women's reproductive lives, concern has been growing among feminists about the autonomy of women in this context. The power of new medical technologies, the cultural epistemic authority of physicians, and the gendered power dynamics in many patient-physician relationships can inhibit women's reproductive freedom. Often those factors interfere with women's ability to trust themselves to choose and act in ways that are consistent with their goals and values. This book introduces to the literature on reproductive ethics the idea that in reproductive health care contexts women's self-trust can be undermined in ways that threaten their autonomy. Understanding the importance of self-trust for autonomy is crucial for understanding the limits on women's reproductive freedom, especially in this age of technological reproduction.

Neither in reproductive ethics nor in bioethics more generally has there been discussion of the value of self-trust for autonomous decision making. Those who have written about trust in bioethics, such as Caroline Whitbeck (1995) and Edmond Pellegrino (1991), refer only to the value of being able to trust our health care providers, given how vulnerable we tend to be as patients. However, in situations of vulnerability it is important not only that we can trust others, but also that we can trust ourselves to stand up for our own interests and for what we value most. Otherwise, we relinquish our autonomy. Thus, having trustworthy professionals is not a solution on its own to patient vulnerability. An important additional element is respect for patient self-trust. This is especially crucial in reproductive contexts, where potential barriers to self-trust among competent patients tend to be greater than in many other health care contexts because of the negative influences that gender oppression and socialization can have on women's reproductive health care choices.

Discussion in theoretical ethics about the importance of self-trust for autonomy is limited; it consists only of Trudy Govier's "Self-Trust, Autonomy, and Self-Esteem" (1993b). Furthermore, the philosophical literature on what self-trust is and how it differs from other self-regarding attitudes is underdeveloped. A lot of theoretical work therefore remains to be done to explain just what it would mean for health care providers to respect the self-trust of their patients and why they have the duty to do so. This book aims to do that work and therefore to contribute not only to the bioethics literature, but also to the philosophical literature on moral psychology.

The theoretical components of the book are grounded in the experiences of some women in the realm of reproductive medicine. Individual cases serve as paradigms illustrating what self-trust is like and why it is important for autonomy. Those cases center around three issues: miscarriage, infertility treatment, and prenatal diagnosis. They come from my own experience doing clinical bioethics in obstetrics, from documentary film, and from sociological and anthropological texts on reproductive medicine.

The treatment that women receive in all areas of reproductive medicine can have a profound effect on what I call their reproductive autonomy. Following Dorothy Roberts, I interpret that term broadly to encompass all procreative activities or events in our lives (1997, 6). Although reproductive autonomy is often understood narrowly in terms of women's civil rights of access to abortion or reproductive technologies, surely the concept should have a wider application. For example, if little respect is given to women's autonomy once they gain access to reproductive technologies, they will lack control over how they reproduce or attempt to reproduce. They will have diminished reproductive autonomy.

The following case illustrates that point and provides insight into the kinds of situations that require patient self-trust. Lee, a nurse and counselor, entered an infertility program feeling confident about where her boundaries lay in terms of how much she was willing to go through emotionally, spiritually, and physically in trying to become pregnant.[1] She left the program feeling powerless and objectified, and as if her identity had been threatened. Such feelings arose largely because of how little control she had over who had access to her body. The program she was in used a team approach in which patients have no guarantees as to who will examine them at any time and who will conduct scheduled procedures. Because of the intrusive nature of physical examinations and procedures involved in infertility treatment, the team approach puts the dignity of women at risk (McLeod and Harris n.d.). As one woman who went through the same program commented, "You park your dignity and integrity at the door and pay this price to get pregnant."

With no real relationship with most of the people treating her, Lee had the impression that she "was only another procedure to be done" or a mere "number . . . in a blood work report." Rarely did anyone address her emotional needs, including the program's counselor. And when Lee tried to advocate for those needs herself, she was labeled "a problem," in her view: another noncompliant patient. The label induced shame about what she described as her "sensitivity" and it made her worry that her care providers would abandon her. Such feelings, together with being treated as a mere object of medical scrutiny, caused her to lose her sense of who she was and of what she needed. Before entering the program she had never thought of herself as uncooperative or as tending to create problems where they do not exist, nor had she ever thought of her body as a mere reproductive vessel to which anyone could have access. In the end, she was left in an extremely vulnerable position.

After Lee left the program she wrote letters to two of the physicians with whom she came in contact. The following is an excerpt from a letter she sent to the physician who gave her a hysterosalpingogram (HSG),[2] and who then performed a hysteroscopy to repair damage to the lining of her uterus that may have been caused by the HSG itself. The excerpt focuses on the events that led up to the hysteroscopy, an experience that Lee described as objectifying. Those events are not isolated, but are rather representative of a larger pattern of unethical patient care.

When you did the informed consent over the phone, I specifically asked you how many people would be in the O.R. [operating room] suite. You told me there would be three people—the anesthetist, the circulating nurse, and yourself. This was a very important issue for me because of my past history of trauma. I don't know if [Dr. X] told you that I originally was asking for spinal anesthesia because I did not want to be unconscious in this type of situation. After talking with the anesthetist and with you over the phone, I felt reassured that I was heard. I couldn't believe when I was wheeled into the room I counted eight people (men and women) there cleaning instruments, laughing and showing no signs of finishing up before you got started (with my entire lower body fully exposed and my legs in stirrups). I looked at you to help me in this and to try to honor my need for control and personal dignity, and you responded in defense of the staff that were cleaning instruments rather than on my behalf. I still remember crying and begging the anesthetist to knock me out because what I was feeling at that moment was unbearable. I now wish that I had gotten up off the table and left the room. . . . It was another episode where I felt objectified.

This situation has a host of ethical problems, not the least of which are the attending physician's disrespect for Lee's earlier requests and his insensitivity to her needs as a woman who had suffered trauma. A less obvious problem, perhaps, is that Lee felt she could not get out of that operating suite and instead had to ask to be "knocked out" by the anesthetist. She was not forced to stay against her will, but she could not muster the will to leave. She could not trust herself to choose and act in ways that were consistent with maintaining her autonomy and dignity.

While the vulnerability Lee felt with her legs in stirrups on the operating room table increased exponentially when she discovered that she could not trust her physician, she was also vulnerable because she was not in a position to be able to trust herself. Why was that the case? One might assume since she was worried about possibly being abandoned that she was simply obsessed with becoming pregnant and thus could not trust herself to act autonomously. However, that stereotype of infertile women is untrue of Lee (and of many infertile women, in fact). Being abandoned was a concern because she wanted to receive *some* treatment and there were no other clinics in her area. Still, she did not have the mindset of doing whatever it takes to fulfil her desire to have a genetically related child. Some factors that explain her lack of self-trust in the operating suite are her objectification as a mere reproductive vessel and shaming by her health care providers, which was related to her "sensitivity," or to what they perceived as her oversensitivity. Such factors are not uncommon in infertility treatment and they are inextricably linked with sexism, as I argue in the feminist bioethical theory of self-trust that

I develop. Such a theory highlights the many obstacles that oppression can pose to the ability of patients to trust themselves.

Women's male partners are certainly not immune to forces that can undermine self-trust in reproductive health care. However, the potential threat to their self-trust is less severe than it is for women either because they are not patients at all or, as in infertility treatment, they are not the patients on whom most procedures and examinations are performed. Furthermore, whereas the gender socialization of men can have a negative influence on their reproductive autonomy (e.g., by persuading them to accept norms that connect masculinity with virility), usually the impact is less severe on men than it is on women. In most societies people tend not to be as suspicious or scornful of adult men who are childless as they are of women who are childless. Hence, I focus my discussion on *women's* self-trust and reproductive autonomy (although I do not ignore the position of their male partners).

The discussion begins with inquiries into the nature of trust and of self-trust. To return to the case of Lee, one might ask why we should identify the barrier to her autonomy as lack of self-trust? Why not lack of self-confidence or of self-respect? Is "self-trust" even meaningful given that we tend to think of trust in interpersonal terms? I take that last worry seriously in chapter 2, and in chapter 3 discuss aspects of self-trust and self-distrust compared with other self-regarding attitudes. Chapter 2 is a conceptual analysis that explains how trust could be self-regarding. By modeling trust on a theory of moral concepts, which states that they are structured by core cases or prototypes, and that we move to less prototypical cases using our moral imagination, we can acknowledge self-trust as a legitimate although nonprototypical variant on trust in others.

In chapter 2, prototypical trust relations such as those between professional and client and parent and child guide us toward a theory of what it is that we trust in others. The literature in bioethics is not particularly helpful on this issue, and the literature in ethics gives inconsistent advice, especially about what kind of motivation we expect people to have in doing what we trust them to do. My theory of interpersonal trust is new to both literatures. Contrary to Annette Baier's highly influential account (1995), I maintain that trust is an attitude of optimism about someone's competence and *moral integrity,* not their competence and *goodwill,* where I interpret "moral integrity" using recent feminist work on the meaning of integrity (Calhoun 1995; Walker 1998).

My theory has important implications for how trust is formed and fostered in relationships. Near the end of the book I recommend how health care providers can promote and preserve patient self-trust in reproductive health care, and I propose that an important part of fulfilling that duty is to establish trust in their relationships with patients. Lee was not able to trust her health care providers to interpret the expression of her needs as legitimate, and as a result, she was not always able to trust herself to act in her own interests. Patients cannot trust themselves to be autonomous if they cannot trust physicians to give them room to express their autonomous desires, and also to inform them accurately about their health and health care options. Patient self-trust does not replace the need for trust between patients and practitioners.

Having learned that trust can be self-regarding, chapter 3 demonstrates that attitudes of self-trust and self-distrust exist. Three biographical sketches illustrate that what some women feel toward themselves before and after miscarriage is analogous to what we feel toward others when we trust or distrust them. Although the women's attitudes do not have all of the important features of interpersonal trust, they have enough so that we would call them self-trust and self-distrust. Prototype theory allows for extending concepts to phenomena that have most, although not all, key features of our prototypes for those concepts.

The cases in chapter 3 reveal how self-trust is distinct from other attitudes of self-appreciation and how it is relational (in the sense of being socially constituted), especially in reproductive health care contexts. For example, pronatalist norms about women's maternal instincts and about maternal self-sacrifice can influence how much a woman trusts herself as to whether she acted responsibly in a pregnancy that ended in miscarriage. Self-trust is an attitude of optimism about our own competence and moral integrity, whereas self-distrust is an attitude of pessimism in that regard. Lee may have felt distrust, rather than merely lack of trust, in her ability to get off that table. She may have been pessimistic either that she was competent to leave—she felt somewhat inert, perhaps, having internalized the objectifying gaze of her health care providers—or that she had the moral integrity to leave and then deal with the shame and possible abandonment that would follow.

Lee's history of trauma made her especially vulnerable to challenges her health care providers posed to her ability to be self-trusting. A different patient, one with a more positive history, could perhaps have dealt with those challenges better, maintaining a firm sense (to quote Lee) of "who she was and of what she needed" in the face of them. With profound and secure self-knowledge, such a patient could probably have trusted herself even without becoming seriously vulnerable. In fact, she would probably be less vulnerable in trusting herself in many situations than she would be in trusting most other people. Whether such ability is a mark of the privilege of having a positive history—that is, of being raised in a supportive social environment where one learns to appreciate oneself and to know oneself well—is my central concern in chapter 4. More generally, that chapter explores the symmetry and asymmetry between self-trust and interpersonal trust on the issue of how vulnerable we are when we trust. One might assume that vulnerability—a key feature of trust—is missing with self-trust, for presumably we should know better what is going on when it is our own selves that we are trusting (Govier 1993b). Are we really that transparent to ourselves, however? Most of us are not, and often the reason has to do with negative social forces, such as oppressive stereotypes or abuse of various degrees, that distort our perception of ourselves. The vulnerability patients incur when trusting themselves is relative, I believe, to the presence or absence of such forces in their lives.

Surely, patients are most vulnerable when they trust themselves too much, in which case their physicians may have to persuade them to trust themselves less (without destroying their self-trust altogether). However, caution is necessary here. Physicians are not always well situated to assess whether patients trust or distrust themselves in justified ways. Whether a particular attitude of self-trust or self-distrust is justified often depends on the sociopolitical position of the subject, which is the central thesis of chapter 5. Physicians must recognize the epistemic limits set by their own social position when they evaluate how well patients trust or distrust themselves.

The theory of the justification of self-trust and self-distrust in chapter 5 is a reliabilist account that is social as well as feminist. The reliabilist part states that we are justified in trusting or distrusting ourselves in a particular domain if we have been reliable in the past in developing, in similar domains, attitudes of self-trust and self-distrust that accurately represent our own competence and moral integrity. The social aspect to the theory emphasizes that it is not only features about *us* that determine whether we have been reliable self-trusters and self-distrusters in the past. Because both attitudes are relational, their reliability depends on the quality of social feedback we receive about them. As we learn from the feminist component of the theory, the feedback is sometimes influenced by sexist, racist, and other oppressive stereotypes about the incompetence and moral inferiority of members of oppressed groups. For example, with Lee, the stereotype that women tend to be overly emotional (and hence morally incompetent), particularly regarding pregnancy, seemed to inform the feedback she received about the trust she placed in her own perception of her emotional needs. Such feedback can interfere with the ability of members of minority groups to develop justified attitudes of self-trust, and consequently it can interfere with their autonomy.

Chapter 6 draws on the theory of justification in chapter 5 to defend the importance of self-trust for autonomy. Not just any self-trust will do; people who consistently trust themselves too much or too little will lose autonomy as a result. Furthermore, too little self-trust or too much self-distrust, even if justified, can inhibit autonomy. Lee was probably justified in trusting herself so little, given how disempowered she was; yet, her self-distrust or lack of self-trust interfered with her autonomy. I develop this theme in chapter 6 and ground it in further cases about women, and men, in infertility treatment.

The position I arrive at in chapter 6—that *justified* self-trust is important for autonomy—raises a number of philosophical concerns. For example, it is unclear what we have to trust well about ourselves to be autonomous. What moral commitments are we optimistic that we will live up to when choosing or acting autonomously? More important, do all forms of autonomy even require such optimism? If that were the case, all autonomous behavior would have to have a moral dimension, which is controversial among philosophers, some of whom wish to distinguish between moral and personal autonomy. In other words, they differentiate behavior in which we act on our moral sense of right and wrong from that in which we aim to satisfy desires that are nonmoral. And they describe both types of behavior using the language of autonomy.

Furthermore, why would trusting ourselves badly diminish our autonomy? It is generally understood in bioethics and moral philosophy that we can make bad choices and still maintain our autonomy (i.e., as long as we are the author of those choices). Can we not trust wrong decisions and still be autonomous? My answer is no, not consistently anyway. Autonomy is not simply about being the author of one's choices. I support a more complex theory than that—one in which autonomy is about directing the path that your life takes—in defining the relations between self-trust and autonomy, and self-distrust and autonomy. I also hold that those relations have important implications for how we think about autonomy. If attitudes of self-trust and self-distrust are relational, or socially constituted, in various ways, autonomy must be similarly relational. My theory builds on accounts of relational autonomy in feminist philosophy according to which sociopolitical relations play an important role in engendering (not only in potentially hindering) our ability to be autonomous (Meyers 1989; Mackensie and Stoljar 2000; Sherwin 1998).

What my theory means for the ethical treatment of patients is the topic of chapter 7. What should health care providers do to ensure that they do not inhibit patients from trusting themselves well? The answer might seem obvious in Lee's case (e.g., do not objectify patients by treating them as though they were "numbers in a blood work report"); however, the answer is not always so obvious. For example, where barriers to patient self-trust are rooted in oppression, what can health care providers do to try to minimize their negative effects? A separate yet equally important question is whether changes are necessary to the whole practice of reproductive medicine, or to the way it is conceptualized, to allow for greater self-trust among patients. Chapter 7 addresses those questions against the background of cases involving prenatal diagnosis, and also in light of earlier cases about infertility treatment and miscarriage. One of my main recommendations is that reproductive medicine should become more woman centred, where "woman" is understood in all of her complexity. When pregnant or during infertility treatment, she has important

needs that are not merely physical; and not uncommonly, she has suffered some severe effects of sexist oppression, including sexual abuse. She
also often possesses valuable knowledge about her own body. Were
greater attention paid to such factors in reproductive medical care, patients would be less vulnerable to harm, as they would be in a better position to trust themselves.

To advocate for such changes, we have to begin at the beginning with
a discussion of what self-trust is and how it relates to interpersonal trust.
We have little choice in the matter because of the dearth of literature in
philosophy on self-trust and confusion concerning the nature of interpersonal trust. Our first task is to try to dispell that confusion.

2

What We Trust in Others: Prototypical Features of Trust

Talk of trust is pervasive in our everyday lives. We commonly hear people ask such questions as "Do I trust my partner?" "Can I trust X [professional person] to do what is in my best interests?" "Do I trust Y well enough to make him responsible for what I care for?" Surely, it is less common to hear "Do I trust myself?" Whereas self-doubt that many people experience may be akin to doubting whether they can trust themselves, we do not easily categorize such attitudes as self-trust or self-distrust. The reason why is that we[1] tend to think of trust in interpersonal terms. In that context, talk of self-trust and self-distrust seems somewhat bizarre.

Whether such talk is even meaningful is open for debate, given that trust, as we understand it, occurs in relationships. Therefore, maybe it does not make sense to speak of trusting the self. People who are plagued with self-doubt simply lack self-confidence or self-respect; it would be a category error to say that they do not trust themselves. Is that true? Is it incoherent to trust the self?

To assume the answer is "yes" on the basis that self-trust is missing one of the salient features of trust (interpersonal relationality) would be to hold too rigid a view of the structure of our concepts. According to a prominent theory of concepts in cognitive science, prototype theory, we can and frequently do extend our concepts beyond the most obvious phenomena that they represent. Many philosophers defend that theory as a plausible account of our *moral* concepts (Johnson 1993; Churchland 1996; Clark 1996; Flanagan 1996). I believe their work is helpful in illuminating how it is that we can conceive of self-trust given the way that we conceive of trust.

To model trust on prototype theory involves taking interpersonal trust to be prototypical and self-trust to be a nonprototypical variant on trust in others. According to the theory, prototypes structure our concepts, which we extend to less prototypical cases depending on their degree of similarity to the prototypes. To know what those less prototypical cases might be, we first must understand the nature of the prototypes. To know what self-trust might be, we first have to understand the nature of interpersonal trust. I use short vignettes to illustrate the kinds of interpersonal relations that inform our concept of trust. Those relations have features in common that explain what it is that we trust in other people, and how, ultimately, trust could be self-regarding.

Thus, my aim is to develop a theory of trust that will allow us to comprehend self-trust. Trust theories in ethics are helpful in this regard, particularly those of Annette Baier (1995) and Karen Jones (1996), both of whom defend a conception of the salient features of interpersonal trusting attitudes. I do not entirely agree with their conclusions, however. Baier's theory, which is highly influential both in theoretical ethics and in bioethics,[2] is flawed in an important respect. And Jones does not correct the flaw, but rather reproduces it in her own work. Baier uses the vague term "goodwill" to describe one of the characteristics that we trust in other people. Guided by my vignettes, I contend that the kind of motivation we expect from people we trust is not goodwill, but moral integrity.

Classical Theory versus Prototype Theory: Understanding Moral Concepts

According to the classical view of concepts in analytic philosophy, what forms their structure is a stable list of necessary and sufficient conditions. Each condition is deemed necessary in the sense that it represents an inherent feature of the phenomenon to which the concept refers. We use the concept appropriately only when all relevant conditions apply. Thus, if interpersonal relationality were a necessary condition of trust, it would be an inherent feature of it, and talk of self-trust would be incoherent. However, there is good reason to reject the classical model; there is good reason to think that our concepts are more malleable than the model allows. An example of a theory that demonstrates their malleability well is prototype theory, according to which our concepts have not a classical structure, but a prototype structure and application beyond standard, prototypical cases.[3]

In interpreting what it means to say that prototypes structure our concepts, the editors of *Mind and Morals: Essays on Ethics and Cognitive Science* remind us to distinguish carefully among prototypes, exemplars, and stereotypes (May et al. 1996, 5). Exemplars are concrete instances of members of a certain conceptual category; for example, any real mother is an exemplar for the category "mother." A stereotype is an exemplar that our culture deems typical of members of the relevant category (e.g., the stereotypical mother). Prototypes, on the other hand, are models that represent different members of a category (not only stereotypical members). To quote Andy Clark (1996, 111), a prototype is "a kind of artificial exemplar that combines the statistically most salient features" of exemplars of the same class to which the subject has been exposed. Since prototypes consist of features that are common within a whole body of exemplars, they are unlikely to match up to any one exemplar. Again, to quote Clark (1996, 111), "the prototypical pet may include both dog and cat features, and the prototypical crime may include both harm to the person and loss of property."

Depending on the nature of the relevant prototypes, applying our concepts to certain exemplars will feel entirely natural. To use an example from Mark Johnson (1993, 78, 80), robin is a "clear, unproblematic case" of bird for many of us in North America. We have no trouble using "bird" to describe robins. When faced with nonprototypical birds, however, such as penguins or emus, we have to extend our concept of bird to them imaginatively. We interpret such odd creatures as birds because they share more of the salient features of our bird prototype than our prototype for other categories, such as mammal, insect, or fish. In this model of concepts, deciding how to conceive of a strange or new phenomenon is a matter of deciding which prototype best characterizes that phenomenon (Churchland 1996, 103).

Our physical and social environments determine what our prototypes will be. And as we come to inhabit new environments, our prototypes will probably change, although only gradually. Say, for example, that I had never been exposed to an environment in which people ascribe moral worth to animals, but then I become immersed in a subculture of vegans and animal rights activists. I will probably experience some change in my prototypes for certain moral concepts, especially rights. It might even become as natural for me to associate rights with animals as it is with humans. Such a shift away from the dominant paradigm of rights in my culture cannot be too radical if I am still to communicate about rights with people in the dominant culture, however. Prototypes can vary only slightly among members of the same cultural and linguistic group, and furthermore, the ideas and experiences of dominant members of the group often have the most profound influence on the nature of our prototypes.[4] Below I illustrate that point using the concept of trust.

Prototype theory is certainly compelling. To use an example in the moral realm, we are not restricted to a list of necessary and sufficient conditions for murder in using the concept "murder." Whereas the voluntariness of the murderer is a key element of that concept, we can imagine an act being murderous if the person acted under duress. Similarly, we can interpret the intentional and brutal killing of an animal as murder, even though the death of a person is the prototype. As long as such acts have enough prototypical features of murder, we would extend the concept accordingly. Therefore, each of those features cannot be necessary. Our concepts are more malleable than traditional analytic philosophy makes them out to be.

However, are concepts such as murder so malleable that *none* of their important features serve as necessary conditions? Surely, an event would not count as a murder unless someone died. A creature would not be a bird if it did not have wings (vestigial or not). Prototype theory states that not every salient feature of our prototypes is necessary, otherwise, the extension of our concepts would be severely limited; yet the theory does not preclude there being *some* necessary features. However, to dwell on that possibility would be to miss the point. What is interesting is the claim that when we apply our concepts to the world, we do not reason from a set of necessary (or sufficient) conditions. We move instead from prototypes to relevant phenomena. And although the move is guided by salient features of the prototypes, it does not occur simply by reasoning from those features.

How do we determine what the salient features of our prototypes are? We picture a certain feature being absent from a clear case in which the concept applies and decide whether the case would still be clear and unproblematic. For example, imagine that robins could not fly. Would we still think of "robin" as a clear case of "bird"? Probably not. Yet what if the feature we had imagined to be missing turned out to be irrelevant to our use of the concept? In that case, the feature must be nonprototypical. Take away the robin's orange belly, would it still be a clear case of "bird"? Yes.

We have a prototype for our concept of trust that is made up of salient features of interpersonal trust relations. I will illustrate what I think are clear, unproblematic cases of trust in Western culture and use them to define what it is that we trust in others in a prototypical sense. Once we sort that out, we can determine whether a self-regarding attitude has enough features of prototypical trust that we would call it self-trust.

Salient Features of Our Trust Prototype

Among the salient features of our trust prototype is clearly interpersonal relationality. Our use of the concept "trust" is not limited to relationships between persons; we often speak of trusting governments or animals, for example. However, in contemplating whether we should apply the concept to those relations, we usually assess whether they are sufficiently similar to interpersonal trust relations. If we were ever truly to evaluate whether we could trust our dog (or someone else's dog), we would consider whether or not features of our attitude toward the dog closely resemble features of the trusting attitudes we have toward other people, such as our best (human) friend.[5] Friendships or intimate relations between persons are usually clear, unproblematic cases of trust in our culture.

Trust is deemed relevant to persons in a prototypical sense; but why not have the relevant person be the self? Cases of self-trust are not clear and unproblematic, perhaps because of the influence of dominant members of our culture on what our prototype is. Prototypes for moral concepts are learned within social environments where some people's experiences (i.e., those of the dominant group) are normalized and other people's are considered aberrant. For people who are not socially dominant, the question of whether they can trust themselves may be common, given how oppressive social forces can undermine one's self-appreciation. Relative freedom from such influences allows many members of dominant groups to take self-trust for granted, to the point that they do not even notice when they do trust themselves. "Do I trust someone else?" seems a more valid question than "Do I trust myself?" because the latter does not figure prominently in the lives of the privileged.

The dominant prototype for trust is therefore interpersonal; but what besides interpersonal relationality are its salient features? Clear cases of trust—what we might call prime exemplars or prototypical relations[6]— should guide us toward an answer. They include child-parent relationships, intimate (and specifically heterosexual[7]) relationships, and professional-client relationships. Each characteristically involves certain kinds of dependency that are indicative of trust (whereas we would not say the same about interactions among strangers, for example). Here are some examples.

Kate is a 9-year-old girl who depends on her father, Stefan, to care for her and to explain things about the world. When she does not understand what her class is learning in school, she relies on Stefan to help her. If she does something wrong, she expects him to be able to tell her why. Stefan speaks with authority on many different issues, and Kate usually assumes that what he says is right.

Mark and Josie are lovers and best friends. They depend on one another for many things, but especially to be loyal, honest, and emotionally supportive. Loyalty and honesty are important to both of them and they know that about each other. They also expect emotional understanding from one another, particularly at stressful times, such as when Mark is fighting with his boss at work or when Josie has a difficult paper to write for graduate school.

For over eight years Todd has had the same family physician, Dr. Young. He has always depended on Dr. Young to provide him with good medical advice and to perform medical procedures competently. He has kept him as his family physician for so long partly because Dr. Young gives him a lot of information about potential harms and benefits of different procedures or treatments. It is important to Todd that he be informed as much as possible about his health care so that he can be sure he truly wants what he is getting.

At least one party in each of these relationships depends on the other in a way suggesting that they have a bond of trust. Kate trusts Stefan's judgment and his concern for her well-being; Josie and Mark trust each other to display certain virtues; and Todd trusts Dr. Young to be a good family physician. These are clear and unproblematic cases in which most of us would not have any difficulty using the term "trust."

I do not mean these to be exemplars of what the different parties should be able to trust in one another. Different people's prototypes for trust will differ depending on what they believe to be essential elements of interpersonal relationships, where what is essential to them will surely depend to some degree on their experience trusting others. For example, if a dishonest partner betrayed me in the past, honesty in new intimate relationship will be particularly important for me. Although it is hard to imagine honesty being irrelevant to someone in an intimate relationship, how relevant it is can vary along with other qualities such as fidelity or modesty, which may not be at all important to some people. I use the vignettes to illustrate only general features of trusting attitudes, those features that the dependent parties must have in common for their relationships to be prime exemplars of trust. Among those features is optimism about the competence of the other in certain domains.

The Competence of the Trusted One
Each dependent party in the vignettes relies on the competence of the other. For example, one thing Kate is optimistic about in terms of her father's competence is his ability to make sound judgments on what is morally right and wrong. Josie and Mark rely on each other to be competent to provide emotional support and to understand what it takes to be a loyal and honest partner. Todd expects Dr. Young to be competent to perform medical procedures and to give Todd sound advice as well as detailed information about his health care options.

If optimism about another's competence were to fade away, so would trust. If Todd were to hear that a number of Dr. Young's former patients were suing him for malpractice and Todd began to seriously doubt Dr. Young's competence as a physician, Todd's trust in him would diminish, if not disappear altogether. If Mark were no longer optimistic that Josie understood what it means to be faithful to him, Mark would no longer trust Josie to the extent that he does.

Sometimes we trust without expecting the other to do something for us, but even there we are optimistic about that person's competence. Most of the characters in the vignettes trust another person to promote their interests in some way or to have specific concern for them. What I call trust with specific concern can be contrasted with trust without specific concern, where we trust someone to do something even though whether or not they do it has no impact on us. An example would be trust in a friend to be conscientious at her work, where the domain of her work does not intersect with our lives. Trust that does not demand specific concern can occur outside of a personal relationship (in which case it is nonprototypical); for example, I trusted Mother Teresa to make truthful statements to others.

Especially in child-parent and professional-client relationships, trusters are often unaware of what the trusted ones have to do to display their competence and the former are vulnerable as a result. For example, Kate trusts Stefan to be competent to make judgments in many areas that Kate knows nothing about. Todd trusts Dr. Young to give him competent advice, even though Todd probably could not tell good medical advice from bad. Some bioethicists emphasize the need for patients to trust their physicians because of the knowledge gap that normally exists between them (Pellegrino 1991; Zaner 1991; Whitbeck 1995). Patients are vulnerable in medical encounters in part because of that gap. Vulnerability is a prototypical feature of trust about which I reserve discussion for chapter 4.

Optimism about the competence of the other in prototypical trust relations is usually domain specific. For example, Todd trusts Dr. Young to have expertise in the domain of medicine, and Josie and Mark trust one another to be competent about certain aspects of intimate relationships. We tend to think that trust between lovers and between a child and a parent is often so comprehensive that it extends to the entire well-being of the trusting person. Still, it is usually not so broad in scope that the truster is optimistic that the trusted is competent at everything. I might trust my mother to be generous and caring toward me, but not trust her to be competent to advise me about my career or how to be a competent canoeist. Even Kate, at her age, probably recognizes that her father has some foibles, such as arriving late for appointments or losing things frequently, making him untrustworthy in certain domains.

Still, one might maintain that it is possible to trust without consideration for domain. We often say that we simply trust someone and do not qualify the statement. Do I not exclude that possibility by describing trust as a four-place relation, of A trusting B to do C in a particular domain D? I do not think so. My logic can accommodate cases where we say that people just trust. There, what they trust other people to do drops out of the picture not because the logic of their attitude is unique, but because there are so many domains in which they trust those people that it is too cumbersome to list them all. They may, in fact, trust them in every domain (in which case their trust would surely be misplaced), or they trust them in a range of domains, the boundaries of which are unclear.

Of interest is that the domains of trust in the vignettes include moral understanding. Such understanding, or knowing what is morally required in different situations, is one dimension of moral competence: the epistemic dimension. Another is acting on what is morally required; that is, being morally virtuous. The latter overlaps with an important feature of trust relations that I discuss: optimism about the moral integrity of the trusted one. Whereas that feature concerns the motivation of people we trust, the epistemic side of moral competence concerns only their ability to understand how they should act.

Jones (1996) noted that the relevant competency in friendships or intimate relations is "a kind of *moral* competence" (her emphasis). "We expect a friend to understand loyalty, kindness, and generosity, and what they call for in various situations" (1996, 7). However, surely that statement needs qualification. First, we do not trust our friends only to possess moral competence. For example, Josie expects Mark to have some idea of the kind of stress she is under as a student, which is a type of nonmoral understanding. Second, we can trust some friends without trusting them to be loyal or generous. Some friends we trust to be generous and caring, others we trust to be insightful and loyal, and so on.

Similarly, trust in parent-child and professional-client relations extends into the moral domain but is not confined to that domain. Kate relies on her father to make competent judgments on many different issues, whether they be moral or nonmoral. With professional people, we rely on their nonmoral understanding (i.e., of their profession). In terms of what moral knowledge we require of them, minimally it tends to include the importance of honoring a commitment to perform some kind of service for us. Nonetheless, from many of them we expect greater moral

understanding than that. For example, Todd is representative of a growing segment of Western society that trusts physicians to understand the
need to respect patient autonomy (along with related issues such as what
counts as justified and unjustified paternalism, and the responsibility of
physicians to disclose information to patients). It is not enough that
health care practitioners have the necessary technical skills and scientific
knowledge to be competent practitioners. Even patients who assume that
physicians should be paternalistic trust physicians to understand the
moral importance of acting in their best interests.

Thus, in the vignettes the truster relies on the trusted to have some
epistemic moral competence. That is part of the more general feature of
optimism about the competence of people we trust to do what we trust
them to do. Our optimism is normally domain specific, which is true even
where our trust does not demand specific concern. For example, my trust
in Mother Teresa extended to her knowledge of the moral importance of
being truthful and caring, particularly for people in desperate circumstances; however, it did not extend to her knowledge of the moral aspects
of abortion.

Motivation of the Trusted One[8]

We want people we trust to have not only the ability to do what we trust
them to do, but also the motivation to do it. Modern trust theory is somewhat confused about what the relevant motivation is. Whereas most
theorists say that it is goodwill, not all trust theorists agree, and some fail
to give a clear answer to the question of motivation.[9] It is important not to
be ambiguous in answering that question because part of what makes
trust different from other attitudes, particularly reliance, is the motivation
we expect from people we trust. I contend that what we expect in prototypical trust relations is moral integrity, where I interpret integrity in light
of philosophical advances in theorizing about it by feminist philosophers
Cheshire Calhoun (1995) and Margaret Urban Walker (1998). Their
work helps us, I believe, to conceptualize trust better.

It cannot only be moral integrity that we demand from people we trust,
however. What moral integrity involves is consistently doing what "one
takes oneself to have the most moral reason to do" (Calhoun 1995, 249).
If what another person's view of what he has the most moral reason to

do frequently differs from what I would take myself to have the most moral reason to do in similar circumstances, I probably would not trust that person. There must be an expectation with trust of some similarity between what we and the trusted person stand for, morally speaking, in the relevant domain.

That expectation plus optimism about the trusted one's moral integrity are further prototypical features of trust relations. I add one other—a feature that concerns the trusted person's perception of our relationship. For us to be optimistic that the other person will be motivated to honor our trust, we have to expect that she shares our view of the nature of our relationship.

Trust and Moral Integrity   Let me begin by proposing that the relevant motivation is moral integrity, not goodwill. Baier and Jones interpret goodwill loosely to mean caring about the good of others or having concern for their welfare (Baier 1995, 102, 136; Jones 1996, 7). They are imprecise about what that concern amounts to: is it kindly or benevolent feeling, which is the vernacular sense of goodwill? Is it a will that is informed necessarily by considered judgments about the other's welfare? If so, are those judgments in some sense moral? If what Baier and Jones mean by goodwill is a kind of moral or just concern for others, their view is not far from my own that what we want from people we trust is moral integrity.

Colloquially, goodwill means kindly feeling toward others. For such feeling to be what we trust in others, it would have to endure to some degree, for we always expect the concern of trusted others to endure, at least over the period of time in which we trust them. Could it be true that what we trust in others is reliable kindly feeling? No, for two reasons: we can trust without expecting people to have kindly feelings for us; and trust can be betrayed when the trusted person is motivated by kindly feelings but does not do the right thing in the circumstances.

We can trust others without being optimistic that they feel kindly toward us, especially when we trust them without expecting them to show specific concern. Whether those whom we trust have feelings or concern for us is irrelevant to our trust in them when our trust does not demand specific concern. Yet even when it does, optimism about their kindly feelings may not be a feature of our trust. For example, it is conceivable that some patients trust their physicians to be motivated by a commitment to provide them with good health care without assuming that the latter have kindly feelings for them. Particularly in trust relations between patients and specialists, such as surgeons, kindly feelings need not be an important part of the relation.

But say that someone did have kindly feelings toward us and they were reliable feelings: would knowing that not be a good reason to trust that person? What if Dr. Young reliably expressed kindly feelings toward Todd? Could Todd not then trust Dr. Young even without knowing whether he was committed to promoting the welfare of his patients? The problem is that Dr. Young could be motivated by such feelings and still betray Todd's trust. Say that not only is Todd optimistic that Dr. Young respects his autonomy, Dr. Young is committed to doing so (where that requires that he disclose information to Todd about his health status and his health care options). If Dr. Young were to develop reliable and kindly feelings toward Todd and be motivated because of those feelings to be dishonest with him about his health status, he would be betraying Todd's trust. He would be failing to inform him of potentially serious health problems, not because he thinks it is his moral duty to prevent Todd from experiencing distress (again, Dr. Young is committed to promoting patient autonomy), but because he has a strong desire not to cause Todd distress. In that case, Dr. Young would be acting on kindly feelings without doing what Todd trusts him to do. Therefore, Todd's trust in him could not be grounded in kindly feelings.

Trust is usually incompatible with serious forms of deception unless deception is necessary to shield the trusting person from severe harm. If Todd became clinically depressed and suicidal, it might be compatible with his trust in Dr. Young for Dr. Young to withhold information from him about a serious illness, at least temporarily. But even where deceiving people is not necessary to protect their welfare, kindly feelings can encourage deception if those feelings are strong enough. What we want, ultimately, from people we trust is not kindly feelings, but commitment to doing what is right in the circumstances. In the scenario above, the right thing for Dr. Young to do, both from his perspective and from Todd's, is to disclose information to Todd in a way that is respectful of his autonomy.

One might claim it is a bit overblown to say that what we want from people we trust is for them to "do the right thing." Maybe we just want them to make considered judgments in determining how best to serve our interests, as opposed to having their kindly feelings motivate them in ways that might subvert our interests. Furthering the good of another often requires that we use our judgment (Baier 1995). This interpretation of goodwill as a component of trust relations is certainly compelling; nonetheless, it fails to capture one aspect of trusting attitudes in proto-typical trust relations. Consider if someone with whom we are in such a relation used his considered judgment to evaluate our interests and acted accordingly, but ignored his responsibilities to others in the process. What if Dr. Young were good at respecting Todd's autonomy, but he also gave preferential treatment to Todd, even over patients who were suffering more than Todd and who had arrived at the physician's office first? Many people in Todd's place would be appalled and insist that was not what they had trusted the physician to do. Presumably, then, I have misconstrued Todd's interests by suggesting that Dr. Young could satisfy them simply by respecting Todd's autonomy. Assuming that Todd is a decent guy, his interest could not be to have others suffer for his own sake. Yet even if he were not a decent guy, it would not be in his interests to see the physician treating patients unfairly; Todd may be disturbed by such treatment if only because it suggests to him that one day Dr. Young might treat *him* unfairly! Either way, what Todd trusts Dr. Young to do is the right thing. He trusts him to be motivated by judgments that are not merely considered but are also moral.

In summary, objections to the idea that we want people we trust to be motivated by goodwill, interpreted as kindly feeling or considered judgment, reveal that what we really want them to be motivated by is moral integrity. We want them to have an enduring commitment to acting in a morally respectful way toward us and we want their actions to accord with that commitment.[10] Having integrity means that your actions are integrated with what you stand for, where having moral integrity means that they are integrated with what you stand for morally. When Dr. Young fails to disclose important information to Todd about his health status, he compromises his moral integrity and in doing so betrays Todd's trust.

The best way to defend that position on trust and moral integrity is to respond to objections, of which there are many. The objections I consider are the following. Having optimism about the moral integrity of people we trust suggests (in light of a common understanding of integrity) that we want them to act as perfect moral agents, which is unrealistic. It implies that we expect them not to be motivated by feelings of affection at all, which seems untrue of many trust relations. The desire to maintain one's moral integrity sounds too self-centred for what we want from people we trust, especially when what we want from them is specific concern for us. Finally, moral integrity is too sophisticated a concept to be what children trust in adults, but the trust of children is surely prototypical.

To reiterate the first objection, relying on people we trust to have moral integrity implies that we expect them never to bow to temptation or pressures from others. But that is too much for what we expect of trusted others. It is common for integrity to be defined in terms of one's ability to resist temptation or challenge, so that the paradigm turns out to be the person who acts on what she stands for without fail. However, that view ignores that we often ascribe integrity to those who "own up to and clean up messes" (Walker 1998, 118); that is, to people who take responsibility when they fail to meet a commitment because they were under too much pressure from others or they experienced some momentary weakness of will. As long as they are accountable for whatever problems they caused, we would still say that they had integrity (Walker 1998). Walker defined integrity "as a kind of reliable accountability"; it concerns how reliable we are in living up to important commitments, but also whether we are willing to be accountable for failing to meet our commitments on some occasions.

Are people who fail to meet their commitments yet are accountable for their actions also trustworthy? That might depend on how often they neglect their responsibilities and create messes for others. Usually we do not conclude after someone breaks a single commitment that he is untrustworthy, unless the relevant commitment is extremely important. If someone regularly fails to honor commitments however, due to temptation, say, or the pressures of everyday life, we would say that he is untrustworthy, even if he does clean up after himself. We would also say that he lacks integrity. People with integrity take their moral commitments seriously, which means that they do not bow to temptation regularly, nor do they regularly make commitments to others that they know they cannot keep.

Although regularly bowing to temptation is inconsistent with having integrity, regularly acting on one's *desires* is not inconsistent with it, as long as those desires are compatible with a commitment to doing what is right. If acting with integrity meant acting solely from the commitment to doing what is right, integrity would not be what many people trust in one another. Intimate partners, such as Josie and Mark, usually trust that the other will act out of feelings of affection rather than out of moral duty. However, people with moral integrity can act out of affection as long as their actions are guided by a commitment to doing what is right. The idea of that commitment playing a regulative function, limiting the sorts of feelings on which we act, comes from Barbara Herman (1981). Herman distinguished between secondary motives, which restrict the ways we act, and primary motives, which provide us with motivation to act.[11] The commitment of a person with integrity to act morally is a secondary motive, regulating her conduct, when it permits her to do what she desires to do. When what she desires to do is something immoral, her commitment to doing what is right takes over as her primary motive and prevents her from acting on that desire. Only when that commitment serves as her primary motive is she forced to act against her immediate desires or feelings of affection. At other times, she can act wholly on such feelings and still have moral integrity.

A further objection to the idea that we want the desire to maintain one's integrity to motivate the actions of people we trust is that it may sound as though we were expecting them to be concerned primarily for themselves (especially if one accepts traditional philosophical accounts of integrity). However, we want the gaze of trusted ones to be set on us, not merely on themselves, particularly in prototypical relations. Traditional theories (Williams 1981, 1973; McFall 1987) described integrity as the virtue of an agent who remains committed to life projects or to whatever values he endorses despite the consequences that might have for others. They suggest, in other words, that integrity is a purely personal virtue of an agent who is able to maintain an integrated self.[12] However, guarding our integrity surely involves more than just guarding our selves from disintegration (Calhoun 1995). Integrity must be a social as well as a personal virtue, because people with integrity "stand for something," and no one stands for anything, only for themselves. They do it "for, and before, all deliberators who share the goal of determining what is worth doing" (Calhoun 1995, 257). In taking a stand, we offer to others our best judgment about how both we and they should live and be treated in our society.

Standing for something involves more than just offering our best judgment, however; and so must integrity, one would think, if it is to count as a social virtue. To support her thesis about the social nature of integrity, Calhoun has to emphasize that in taking a stand, we take some responsibility for ensuring that what we stand for is preserved or established. That kind of responsibility is "forward-looking" (Card 1996), whereas reliable accountability is often merely "backward-looking."[13] Since integrity involves responsibilities that move in either direction, a person with integrity cannot be self-indulgent or merely self-protective.

The view that integrity involves forward- and backward-looking responsibilities allows us to make sense of how a child could trust in another person's moral integrity. One might assume that, especially for children younger than Kate (say 5 or 6 years old), moral integrity could not be what they trust in their parents. And since parent-child relations are clearly prototypical of trust, I must have it wrong about the relevant motivation in trust relations. However, consider how someone could trust in another's moral integrity without having a sophisticated understanding of the concept of integrity. A child who trusts her parents to care for her and to make things right when things go wrong trusts them to fulfill forward- and backward-looking responsibilities. Hence, she trusts their moral integrity.

Those who act with moral integrity act on what they take to be the best moral reasons for everyone to act; however, they do not necessarily act on reasons that are morally correct. Having integrity in general "hinges on acting on one's own views, not the right views (as those might be determined independently of the agent's own opinion)" (Calhoun 1995, 250). Integrity is about personal integration, not only social responsibility; and therefore, to have integrity, it is crucial that people act on values that *they* endorse. Nonetheless, minimal substantive restrictions may exist on what values a person with *moral* integrity can endorse. We tend not to recognize vicious dictators or serial killers as having moral integrity. However, we can conceive of people whose moral values are somewhat different from ours as having integrity on the assumption that every moral value of our own may not be entirely objective. Uncertainty surrounding our own moral values allows us to acknowledge moral integrity among people with whom we disagree morally to some degree. We accept that what it means for them to act on their moral values is the same as what it means for us to act on ours.

What the Trusted One Stands For   Because people with moral integrity do not necessarily agree on what is right, it cannot just be moral integrity that we expect from those we trust. We care about *what* they stand for, not just about whether they will act on it. Todd does not trust Dr. Young simply to act on whatever values Dr. Young accepts as right ones. Todd expects him to endorse specifically the value of respect for patient autonomy. In trusting Josie, Mark cares not only about whether she intends to live up to her commitment to him, but also how she conceives of that commitment. He expects Josie to share with him a commitment to being emotionally supportive, loyal, and honest in intimate relationships. If he did not expect that, he undoubtedly would not trust her as an intimate partner. I contend that a further feature of prototypical trust is an expectation that what the trusted person stands for morally speaking is similar enough to what we stand for (as far as we know what that is) that we can count on that person to do what we trust her to do.

To trust others usually we require some sense of what they stand for so that we can know whether they are likely to act in the way we would expect them to. The way we expect them to act depends on what we perceive to be morally acceptable ways to act. What Josie expects from partner she trusts is loyalty and honesty because she believes those are important in intimate relationships. Still, to say that she simply expects loyalty and honesty is vague, since she may not trust a lover who defines loyalty as avoiding all conversations with people to whom one might be sexually attracted. We have to know enough about how people we trust conceive of their moral commitments that we can count on them in certain ways. And since we usually trust others to behave in certain ways only within particular domains, what is most important is that we know where they stand in the domain where we trust them.

One might ask whether it is at all realistic that we require an idea of where people stand, morally speaking, before we trust them. Do we not sometimes trust without knowing ahead of time whether people are committed to acting in the ways we think they should in relevant circumstances? What about when we accept the help of a stranger when our groceries have fallen all over the street? We generally do that sort of thing easily without being aware of what the other person stands for. Would we actually trust the stranger, though, if we assumed that he would probably steal our groceries or beat us over the head while we were bending down to pick them up? No. But how could we assume anything about where his moral commitments lie if we have never met him before? The answer is that it is reasonable for us to assume that other members of our society share at least some values with us. If we could not make that assumption, because either we knew that we were wildly eccentric or we were recent immigrants to this country and were uncertain about which values people held in common here, we would have a lot of difficulty trusting other people.

What if someone did not know whether she should trust others not because of cultural difference, but because she is uncertain about what she herself stands for? What about young Kate, who might stand for some things, but not enough that she knows how she should expect people to act in many circumstances. Would it be possible for her to be trusting in those circumstances? Presumably, without knowing what she should expect, she would not be able to figure out whether she should trust people given what they stand for. Nonetheless, if she admired what they stood for, generally speaking, could she not trust them even without having specific expectations regarding their behavior? Kate could trust her father in that way if she admired him (which she certainly seems to do). By "admiration," I mean simply looking up to another, which is something a younger child than Kate could do. Small children tend to look up to their parents and rely on them to be caring. And in doing so, they express what is akin to admiration for their parent's values.

An adult who is uncertain about what she values in a particular context could trust someone whose judgment she admires. A pregnant

woman who admires her obstetrician's judgment could trust her to decide what is best with respect to prenatal diagnosis, for example, even if
she has no idea what her own values concerning that option should be.[14]
There, she would trust the obstetrician, not because what they both stand
for is relevantly similar, but because what the obstetrician stands for is
presumably consistent with what she would hope to stand for in that
context.

One might object that in these examples admiration for the other's
values is a *consequence* of trusting, rather than something that makes
trust possible. The child admires his parent's judgment and the patient
admires her physician's *because* trust is present in their relationships.
However, we have no reason to presume that admiration could not pre-
cede trust or that trust and admiration could not develop simultaneously
and exist in equal degrees. What I called admiration may grow or diminish alongside of trust in children's relationships with their parents,
for example.

Thus, an expectation about or admiration for what people stand for
morally speaking is an important element of prototypical trust relations.
One could add that our trust in those relations tends to grow or diminish as our knowledge of what the other stands for increases. Furthermore, the amount of evidence we require about how similar their values
are to our own will depend on what is at stake for us in trusting them.
For example, there is more at stake in trusting a lover to move in with
us than there is in trusting one to stay overnight twice a week. Presumably, we would want to know more about our lover's values in the first
case than we would in the second before trusting that person.

But what if we could guarantee somehow that our lover's values were
the same as ours without relying on that person's moral integrity? Could
we not then trust our lover? What about abusive relationships, in other
words, in which one party manipulates the other into holding distorted
views of love and loyalty? Mark could coerce Josie into believing that
loyalty to him involves never speaking to other men so that he could rely
on her to be committed to such "loyalty." In that case Mark does not expect Josie to act on what she stands for (i.e., to act with moral integrity);
rather, he relies on her to act on what he himself stands for. But if that
were so, would we still want to say that Mark *trusts* Josie?

Trust versus Mere Reliance   When we expect people to act in certain ways only because they have been coerced or because they have a non-moral disposition to so act, we are merely relying on them, rather than trusting them (Baier 1995).[15] Reliance is an attitude toward another person's competence where, as long as that person is motivated to do what she is competent to do, it is irrelevant to us what kind of motivation she has for acting. Hence, reliance can be compatible with sleazy motives (hostility, hatred), with motives that are morally indifferent, or with positive motives, including moral integrity. Thus, I assume that trust is a form of reliance. Cases of mere reliance are those in which we are optimistic that the other will act from a motive other than moral integrity. For example, I might be optimistic that a surgeon will perform surgery competently not because I believe he has any moral integrity, but because I know he does not want to be sued.[16] There, the language of trust would be out of place, although not because I would necessarily behave differently with the surgeon who fears social sanctioning as opposed to the one who acts with moral integrity. I might be willing to put my life in the hands of either surgeon as long as they were equally competent.

So what is the difference between such cases? According to Richard Holton (1994), when we expect people to act purely out of selfishness or out of duress, we do not trust them, for we would not feel betrayed if they failed to do what we relied on them to do. We would feel betrayed, however, if we had trusted them to do it. Feeling betrayed is the expected emotional response to broken trust; and it is not a feeling we would have toward people on whom we had merely relied. For Holton, what is special about trust, compared with reliance, is that when we trust, we adopt a stance of readiness to feel betrayed.

However, I question whether such a stance of readiness alone could be what distinguishes trust from reliance. The response of betrayal is a negative moral assessment of the behavior of others relevant specifically when they fail to honor commitments that we trusted them to meet. If they do not do what we trusted them to do through no fault of their own, we would not say that they betrayed us. Since betrayal has a moral element to it, feelings of betrayal are appropriate only toward people whom we expected to act morally. Thus, what makes trust different from reliance is not merely, or even ultimately, that betrayal is specific to broken trust.

Trust and reliance are distinct because we expect people we trust, unlike those on whom we merely rely, to be motivated by a moral commitment.

Given the prototype structure of trust and reliance, we should assume not that those attitudes are entirely distinct, however, but that they lie on a continuum. Clear cases of trust are those in which we expect the trusted one to be motivated primarily by a moral commitment. But in less prototypical cases we accept that the other will probably act on some nonmoral or even immoral desire as well. The thought that such a desire might be present together with moral concern does not preclude our attitude about trust.

Of course, we can trust someone who intends to act purely out of sleazy motives as long as we are unaware of that fact. Our trust would simply be misplaced. Where the trusted one lacks integrity and relies on the "successful cover-up of breaches of trust" to keep the trust relation going, trust is in the relation but it is "morally rotten" (Baier, 1995, 255).[17] Not all trust theorists agree on that point, however. Jones (1996) and Judith Baker (1996) assume that trust requires not only optimism that the trusted one will be concerned for our welfare, but actual concern for our welfare. When people we trust rely on concealment of breaches of trust, their relationship with us is one of reliance, not trust (Jones 1996, 19). Trust, like friendship, is a relation that one party can destroy by being deceitful even if the other party is not aware of the deceit (Baker 1996). Jones and Baker focus on a specific way in which we use the term trust. We often say that trust is missing from a relationship when one party is deceiving the other successfully. But do we really mean that no trust of any kind is left in the relationship? We would still say that the duped party *trusts* the other party, would we not? An adequate theory must make room for misplaced trust.

One can also trust and be wrong about similarities between what the trusted person stands for and what one stands for, or would hope to stand for. For trust to thrive, it is important only that one's expectation about those similarities persist, and, of course, that one remains optimistic about the moral integrity and competence of the other person.

The Trusted One's Perception of our Relationship   A further feature, one that is relevant only to prototypical relations, is that we expect people we trust to interpret the nature of our relationship similarly to the way we do. If they conceive of our relationship differently, they may not welcome our trust. Adding that feature takes care of unwelcome trust (a problem raised in the literature by Karen Jones), and it concerns our attitude specifically toward *whether*, as opposed to *how*, people we trust will be motivated to act.

When people do not welcome our trust, they do not object to our optimism about their competence, their moral integrity, or about the fact that we admire what they stand for. Rather, according to Jones, they object to our expectation that they do something for us (1996). That is an objection to the idea that they be "directly and favourably moved by the thought that we are counting on them" (Jones 1996). Jones defined that expectation as a feature of all trust relations partly as a way to solve the problem of unwelcome trust.[18] However, to assume it is a feature of all such relations is to ignore that we do not always count on people we trust to do something for us. Furthermore, when we do rely on them to show specific concern for us, we do not always expect them to acknowledge our trust and be favorably moved by it. Surely, I can trust that what motivates some people to act respectfully toward me is their own moral sense rather than my trust in them.

The problem of unwelcome trust can arise only when we trust people to have specific concern for us. Let us consider that kind of trust in more detail. How does optimism about people's moral integrity translate into an expectation, in some cases but not others, that they will behave in certain ways toward us? It does so only if the moral commitments on which we expect them to act require them to promote or respect our interests. Whereas some moral commitments demand that we respect the interests of everyone (e.g., our duty not to commit murder), others require only that we behave in a certain way toward people with whom we are in a special kind of relationship. Although I may have a duty to be honest on some level with everyone, I am not morally required, I do not think, to be as honest about my feelings with everyone as I am with people with whom I am intimate. Similarly, I am not morally obligated to be as concerned for the welfare of others as I ought to be for my own family members and close friends. Often what we trust in others, including parents, lovers, and professional people, is that they do something for us that they would not do for just anyone. In other words, we trust them to act on relationship-specific commitments.

Unwelcome trust is a potential problem only in relationships where one expects the other to have what I call *special* concern, which is a factor in all prototypical trust relations. When we trust others to have specific concern that they are committed to having toward everyone, unwelcome trust should not be an issue. If we trust them to have special concern, that is, to do only what they are committed to doing in certain kinds of relationships, our trust might be unwanted. It would be unwanted, specifically, if we expected the trusted person to interpret our relationship differently from the way she does. For example, if a student trusts his teacher to be emotionally supportive in the way that a parent would be, but the teacher does not (nor does she want to) think of her relationship with the student as being like that, the student's trust would be unwanted. Yet by having such trust in his teacher, the student must expect her to think of their relationship as more like a parent-child relationship than a teacher-student one. Without that expectation, he could not be optimistic that she would be emotionally supportive in the way that she would with her own child.

Dealing with unwelcome trust in prototypical relations by including the expectation about how the other perceives our relationship also allows us to explain some cases in which trust is unwelcome but is nonetheless justified. A person who is not favorably moved by my trust might have encouraged me to have expectations that are appropriate only to the kind of relationship *I* think we have. That person does not welcome my trust, but he *should* welcome it because my perception of our relationship is accurate.

Conclusion

With that last expectation, we come to a rather complex understanding of what trust is prototypically. Aside from interpersonal relationality, trust has prototypical features that include optimism about the trusted person's competence and moral integrity in certain domains, together with two expectations, which concern what that person stands for and her perception of our relationship. That analysis might seem so complex as to be implausible, given how pervasive trust is and how easily some of us seem to trust other people. However, it is important to recognize that a trusting attitude (and each feature of it) need not be conscious for trust to exist. Because trust *is* so pervasive—we trust people in so many ways every single day—"such a thing as unconscious trust" (Baier 1995, 99) must exist.

We are most conscious of what the key elements of trust are when some of those elements are missing. If we felt pessimistic, rather than optimistic, about someone's competence and moral integrity, we would not trust that person, but would rather distrust him. Distrust differs from trust in being an attitude of pessimism rather than optimism about the competence and motivation of the other (Jones 1996, 7). Furthermore, if we suspected that someone did not have certain values in common with us or did not share our perception of our relationship, we probably would not trust that person. Note that *not* trusting is not the same as *dis*trusting. Trust and distrust are "contraries but not contradictories, for one may fail to trust without actively distrusting—one may simply not adopt any attitude at all toward the goodwill and competence of another" (Jones 1996, 15, 16). One might feel that another person's values are offensive but have no occasion to trust that person and so not actually *dis*trust him.

It is possible that we have a prototype for distrust as well as trust, and if so, we would classify the exemplars of those attitudes as more or less trusting or distrusting depending on how similar they are to both prototypes. Attitudes can differ in the degree of optimism or pessimism they entail, and hence trust and distrust must admit of degrees.

We know therefore that trust and distrust are particular forms of optimism and pessimism and that trust has many prototypical features. The question now is whether a self-regarding attitude exists that has enough of those features to qualify as a nonprototypical variant of trust. Furthermore, if such an attitude exists, how is it especially relevant to women's reproductive health care as opposed to other attitudes that are self-regarding? In the next chapter I explore those issues from within the context of miscarriage.

3
What We Trust in Ourselves: A Contextual Analysis

Women tend to experience a myriad of self-regarding emotions during pregnancy and miscarriage. Choices surrounding pregnancy and the loss of choice when a pregnancy ends abruptly can call into question one's gender identity, which for many women is intimately bound up with their competency as mothers and their commitment to motherhood. In acknowledging how emotionally challenging those experiences can be, the literature on women's reproductive health often refers to women's self-confidence or lack of it, their self-respect or lack of it in reproductive contexts. One self-regarding attitude that the literature tends to overlook completely is self-trust or the lack of it. That attitude is distinct from self-confidence and self-respect, and I maintain that it describes more accurately some self-regarding emotions that women feel during pregnancy and miscarriage. The importance of noticing that fact lies in the distinct role that self-trust plays in autonomous decision making. In recognizing that what some women feel toward themselves after miscarriage is self-distrust, we can determine how their autonomy may have suffered because of that experience.

Since some might question whether self-trust and self-distrust are meaningful attitudes, I say that they are meaningful and theorize about their nature using the theory of trust I developed in chapter 2, together with sketches of some women's experiences with miscarriage. Developing a theory of self-trust in the context of miscarriage confirms the relevance of that theory to reproductive ethics. It also permits some exploration into the ethical duties that practitioners have toward women and their partners after miscarriage.

The topic of miscarriage has received barely any attention in bioethics, which may seem appropriate given how "nature" has conveniently resolved the potential messy dilemmas of pregnancy that we often discuss in reproductive ethics. But moral issues arise for the reproductive health care of women who have miscarried, and our lack of attention to them seems to reflect greater attention generally (especially among nonfeminists) to the welfare of fetuses compared with that of the women. With the death of the fetus comes the end of our moral deliberations. What we ignore by stopping there is the profound effect that sensitivity (or insensitivity) of health care providers toward the grief or loss that often accompanies miscarriage can have on how women and their partners deal with it (Lasker and Toedter 1994). By their reactions, health care practitioners can either enhance or minimize the self-distrust that can plague these women.

But to know what kinds of reactions can cause or promote self-distrust and consequently threaten women's reproductive autonomy, we must know more about what self-distrust and self-trust are. If health care providers have an obligation to respect the ability of patients to trust themselves enough to get through difficult experiences such as miscarriage, they must understand the nature of self-trust. Advice to providers that they should preserve trust either from patients or of patients toward themselves is basically empty without some description of that attitude. Knowing what it means to trust someone or to trust oneself is crucial for knowing how to enhance trust.

Self-Trust as a Nonprototypical Variant on Trust in Others

To understand self-trust, we first have to understand interpersonal trust. Previously, I modeled trust on a prototype theory of concepts,[1] according to which self-trust could only be a nonprototypical variant of trust in others. Interpersonal trust is prototypical, and self-trust, if it is coherent, must share many of its salient features. Two of those features are optimism about the competence of trusted others and optimism about their moral integrity. When we trust physicians, we trust that they will be competent to care for us and essentially that they will respect us enough to be committed to our care. Moral philosophers and bioethicists tend to agree that trust is a moral attitude, which is what distinguishes it ultimately from reliance. Distrust differs from trust in being an attitude of pessimism rather than optimism about someone's competence and moral integrity.

As I stated at the end of chapter 2, we also expect that those whom we trust share similar values with us, particularly values that are relevant in the domain of our interaction with them. We can be optimistic that physicians will fulfill certain professional duties (e.g., act in our best interests, respect our autonomy) only if we also expect them to have those commitments. And since some moral commitments are relevant only to certain kinds of relationships, we also have to be able to expect that people we trust perceive their relationship with us similarly to the way we do. Moral commitments of physicians to their patients extend neither to the patients of other physicians nor to every patient who walks through the door necessarily (unless one is unfortunate enough to be the only physician on call). An implicit expectation with our trust in certain physicians is that they acknowledge us as *their* patients; that is, as patients with whom they have a certain moral relationship.

That last component of trust is clearly absent in the case of self-trust. The issue does not arise there of what kind of relationship exists between the truster and the trusted. Self-trust is missing the feature of interpersonal relationality, which is why its coherence is in question. Trust might be inherently relational in the sense that it never occurs outside of a relationship between two distinct entities. Although prototype theory allows that some features of our prototypes might be necessary, it is not clear why that would be true of the relationality of trust. Whereas optimism about the trusted one's moral integrity could be necessary because it distinguishes trust from reliance, interpersonal relationality does not obviously serve a similar purpose.

Self-trust may not be relational in the sense of embodying two entities in relation, but it is relational in a different sense, one that becomes obvious when we consider the harmful effects that a health care provider's insensitivity can have on the way a woman feels toward herself after miscarriage. Self-trust and distrust are relational in being socially constituted. They are molded to a significant degree by the responses of others and by societal norms. I devote the end of this chapter to an investigation of their social nature.

Right now we must be get clear on whether self-trust has enough other features of trust, besides interpersonal relationality, to be a meaningful attitude. And if it is meaningful, what is it like compared with interpersonal trust? Furthermore, how can we identify whether a person trusts or distrusts herself, which is a question of some relevance to health care providers if they have a duty to preserve or bolster patient self-trust? Let me provide a specific example of a woman who described certain self-regarding attitudes she had before and after miscarriage that I think are instances of self-trust and self-distrust.

Janet miscarried her first child at seven and a half weeks' gestation. To conceive it, she and her partner, Richard, had "charted and monitored [her] cycle with great care until the exact moment" that they knew she could conceive. All along, Richard was intimately involved in that process. Firm believers in natural family planning, he and Janet had used natural methods of contraception, which made them very familiar with her cycle. When Janet became pregnant, her charts showed it and her physician accepted them as evidence (Hey et al. 1996, 42).

Here is an excerpt from what Janet wrote about the miscarriage and more specifically about her interaction with her physician:

Every morning the bleeding stopped and every afternoon it started and on the Wednesday we went back to our doctor. He felt, palpated, and prodded and questioned that I had ever been pregnant at all: "You told me you were pregnant and I believed you." And I, knowing that I had been pregnant, started to doubt myself and my knowledge of my body. I felt concerned for the doctor, that he felt he had made a mistake, and it was my fault. You are very willing to believe that everything is your fault. . . . I was afraid that the whole episode had just been hysteria, and he (the GP) was thinking "neurotic woman." . . . [She then explained that she had an ultrasound which confirmed her pregnancy.] . . . I had known that I was pregnant, and I had doubted it, doubted me, doubted this little baby's existence because some forms of knowledge are seen as more valid than others. (Hey et al. 1996, 44, 45)

It is not uncommon for women who miscarry to say that they knew they were pregnant but their doctors doubted it. Pregnancy tests early in the first trimester can be unreliable[2]; before the ultrasound, Janet had two such tests and both were negative. Her doctor assumed that she was having a late menstrual period.

Janet expressed self-regarding attitudes that have to do with her knowledge of her pregnant state. Before the physician questioned her judgment about being pregnant, she was certain that it was correct: she mentioned "knowing I had been pregnant," and "my knowledge of my body." There, she assumed some expertise on her part in recognizing changes in her body, specifically, changes that occur in pregnancy. As I acknowledge below, she could easily have been wrong in that assumption, especially since she had never been pregnant before. We are given no information as to why she thought she knew what being pregnant feels like. Perhaps she had learned so much from other women or from books that she could identify the relevant bodily changes. I do not presume that Janet's "knowledge of her body" is privileged, and hence, that her physician's comment "You told me you were pregnant and I believed you" was inappropriate insofar as it challenged her claim (although I do think it was inappropriate for other reasons).

When Janet's physician denied that she had been pregnant, she began to distrust is herself. She did that for two reasons. One is that she may have been wrong to assume that she had the expertise to make that kind of claim; as she said, she "started to doubt . . . [her] knowledge of [her] body." That feeling arose because the physician contradicted her and she assumed that his expertise was greater than hers. Influencing that assumption was an ideological norm favoring knowledge that is grounded in technical scientific evidence rather than in nontechnical evidence that cannot always be verified by standard scientific methods (the former are what Janet referred to as "forms of knowledge [that] are seen as more valid than others"). For a while, Janet accepted that her physician had greater expertise than she did because he was trained to access evidence of pregnancy that is technical, whereas her alleged expertise was informed in part by experiential evidence (or what she perceived to be evidence). She had some technical evidence drawn from her basal temperature charts, but much of the information she relied on came from her own bodily experience (she referred to her knowledge of her body).

Janet also questioned her claim because she wondered whether it could have been motivated by hysteria. Perhaps it was prompted, in other words, by an obsession she had with wanting to have children, and because of that desperate need she deceived herself about whether the evidence pointed, in fact, to pregnancy. The physician's comment encouraged her to question her motivation; it conveyed to her the sexist attitude that women are simply prone to wishful thinking or to being overly emotional. As soon as Janet suspected that her claim was false, she began to feel guilty because she had persuaded the doctor to believe it and as a result, she may have caused him to make a mistake.

Given Richard's involvement in charting Janet's cycle and deciding whether she was pregnant, it may seem unreasonable that Janet took full responsibility for that decision. The alleged mistake was not entirely hers, it was also Richard's (although, of course, Janet alone was responsible for claiming to have embodied knowledge of pregnancy). But as Janet says, "you are very willing to believe everything is your fault." Often, where that comes from is the societal norm that women alone (as opposed to women and their partners) are responsible for what happens during pregnancy. Janet's doctor confirmed that expectation when he said, "*you* [rather than you and Richard] told me that you were pregnant and I believed *you*," even though Richard was present at appointments with the physician. Whether the physician believed Richard was irrelevant, presumably, because it was Janet's responsibility to tell him the truth.

I think Janet trusted herself to tell the doctor the truth before her miscarriage, and afterward, she distrusted her judgment. The self-regarding emotions she felt mimic the kinds of trusting attitudes we have toward others when we rely on their knowledge or expertise. Just as we are optimistic about the epistemic competence of health care providers when we trust them to give us accurate information about our health status, Janet was optimistic that she was competent to inform others about her pregnant state. Her self-trust disappeared after the doctor reprimanded her for supposedly giving him false information.

For Janet's attitudes to be self-trust and self-distrust, however, they would have to target more than just her epistemic competence in the domain of her pregnancy. She would also have to feel some optimism or pessimism about her moral integrity in that domain; otherwise, her attitudes would be indistinguishable from mere reliance. For trust and distrust to remain distinct from reliance, they cannot be so malleable that the moral component drops out completely. (Although that feature may seem absent when we "trust" something like a computer, in such cases, we are probably anthropomorphizing the entities we trust, assuming they could have moral or immoral intentions toward us. We must be thinking that the computer that crashes deserves our moral disdain as we yell at it and smash the keys in anger and frustration!)

So for Janet to have been trusting herself, she must have been optimistic that she would live up to a certain moral commitment; yet what could that commitment have been? I think it was to be honest about what she knew, or, in more sophisticated terms, to be epistemically responsible. Sexist norms denying that women tend to be responsible in that sense (rather than engaged, e.g., in wishful thinking) are hostile to women's moral integrity. People who are responsible epistemically have no intention of deceiving others or deceiving themselves by making false or exaggerated claims. They are committed to telling to truth, as opposed to telling people what they want to hear. They are careful in assessing whatever evidence they have available and furthermore, they willingly accept the limits to their knowledge (i.e., that what they know is limited by whatever they have actual evidence to support).

But it is not only the bounds of evidence that determine epistemic responsibility; it is also what counts as evidence, which is often partly a political issue. Sometimes, dominant groups gain the power that knowledge brings by ensuring that whatever is considered evidence is whatever they have expertise in assessing,[3] and they control who develops that expertise. They exact limits on who gets to be epistemically responsible by promoting a narrow conception of evidence. It seems obvious that Janet did not endorse the dominant conception of evidence in medical contexts, a conception that devalues forms of knowledge the less technical they are. The standard of epistemic responsibility informing whatever commitment she had to tell her physician the truth must have been a revised version of the dominant standard.

Did Janet have that commitment or not? Was she concerned yet optimistic that she was being responsible in telling the doctor that she was pregnant? Some evidence that she had been optimistic is her fear that the "whole episode had just been hysteria." She had not pictured herself as a woman obsessed, rushing to her physician with only the tiniest bit of evidence that she might be pregnant.

What about the guilt Janet suffered after she became suspicious of her knowledge of her body? That seems to be a response to the trust her physician placed in her, but might it also have been a response to broken self-trust? In fact, those two affective attitudes of trusting oneself and of welcoming the trust of others are often closely intertwined. In accepting the trust that others have in us, it is appropriate that we be self-trusting, that we trust that we have the competence and moral integrity to do what they trust us to do. In being optimistic about her ability to know whether or not she was pregnant, Janet would have been trusting herself to live up to certain expectations of people around her, including the physician. But, surely, she would have trusted herself for her own sake as well, since her emotional well-being was at stake. The moral commitments of self-trusters can be self-directed or other-directed; Janet's probably would have been both.

The question of whether or not Janet's guilt is a sign that she had trusted herself is complicated for a number of reasons. The connection between feelings of guilt and broken self-trust is not straightforward, yet it is worth exploring, and not only to be able to establish that attitudes like Janet's are real instances of self-trust and self-distrust. Understanding that connection puts us in a better position to detect whether a person has lost self-trust, which is something for which others might be morally responsible. Health care providers who cause their patients to lose self-trust by being insensitive or domineering are morally responsible, I think, to make amends. They have to allow their patients to be self-trusting again in interactions with them. But they also must have some idea of when they might have made that moral mistake.

Expected Emotional Responses to Broken Self-Trust

How do we know whether a person's self-trust has been shattered? How do we identify broken self-trust? Often we notice that interpersonal trust has been broken when feelings of betrayal surface. It is clearer than ever that we have destroyed the trust of a friend or a lover when we realize that he has such feelings. Feeling betrayed is the expected emotional response to broken interpersonal trust from the one trusting. However, with self-trust we are also the one trusted. We were counting on ourselves to be trustworthy when we betray our trust in ourselves, and hence, one would expect us to respond as the trusted person would when interpersonal trust is broken. What is the expected emotional response there? How does one feel, in other words, when one fails to honor the trust of another? The answer is guilt or, alternatively, shame.

I said that Janet felt guilty when she worried that she might have been playing the role of the neurotic woman; however, it is likely that she felt shame as well. In the philosophy of emotions, the two are distinguished from one another by associating guilt with our actions and shame with our nature (Bartky 1990; Deigh 1983). We feel the betrayal of broken self-trust more deeply when we respond with shame, for in that case betrayal represents not only a wrongdoing on our part, but a shortcoming, a flaw in our character (Bartky 1990, 87). Since wrongdoings usually reflect badly on our character, shame and guilt often accompany one another. Yet, "the boundaries between them tend to blur in actual experience. Psychological studies have shown that most people are hard put to state the difference between shame and guilt, nor can they easily classify their experiences under one heading or the other" (Bartky 1990, 87, 88; see ftn 23 citing Miller 1985). Janet felt guilty about possibly misleading people (including herself, perhaps), but she also might have felt ashamed for seeming neurotic or hysterical.

Thus, one indication of whether a patient's self-trust has been destroyed is that she feels shame or guilt. However, it is only an indication. People can feel guilty or ashamed about their behavior even though they never actually trusted themselves to behave differently. Sometimes we have those feelings, for example, when we fail to live up to certain standards even though we had only been hopeful that we would live up to them. Consider that I made a New Year's resolution to exercise more often. But I never really took seriously the possibility that I would do that, knowing how lazy I tend to be about exercising. So I was hopeful, and I probably felt guilty, even ashamed perhaps, when I returned to my slovenly ways after the holidays. But one would not go so far as to say that I had trusted myself to exercise.

One might suspect that Janet was hopeful rather than optimistic that she was competent to tell her doctor that she was pregnant, since she had never been pregnant. How could she have been optimistic without prior knowledge of pregnancy? However, that question is more about whether she might have been *justified* in trusting herself, rather than about whether she actually trusted herself. Janet could have possessed self-trust, but it was unjustified.

One could feel guilty or ashamed about failing to meet a standard of good behavior even though at the time one was neither optimistic nor hopeful that one would live up to it. That would have been the case with Janet if she had suspected all along that her claim to be pregnant was false, but had encouraged the physician to believe it. That version of her story is not very plausible. Her narrative gives no indication of a conscious intention to deceive, but every indication that she truly believed in her pregnancy.

A final alternative in assessing Janet's negative feelings toward herself is that she internalized the standard that she felt guilty for violating, but she never actually accepted that standard, and hence, was never optimistic that she would live up to it. She did not believe that technical, scientific evidence is inherently superior to experiential evidence; but still, that societal epistemic norm might explain some of her guilt. After the physician questioned her, Janet might have thought (however briefly) that she should never have given as much weight as she did to the evidence she presumed to have. But she could have thought that without actually believing it, that is, without endorsing the dominant standards on evidence, if she had internalized those standards to some degree. Guilt or shame in response to internalized norms does not signal prior optimism about acting with moral integrity, since integrity is about acting in accordance with standards that we accept.

All of that is to say that Janet's guilt or shame does not necessarily indicate broken or damaged self-trust. To show that she had been optimistic about her moral integrity or, more specifically, about her commitment to tell her physician the truth, we must have further evidence. Does her story provide any? I think it does in her statement that she and Richard had "charted and monitored [her] cycle *with great care* until the exact moment" that they knew she could conceive (my emphasis). That Janet took such care reveals that she was committed to acting responsibly and, moreover, that she was optimistic (rather than hopeful but never actually serious) that she was being honest regarding her claim. That evidence, together with the emotional response of guilt and shame, strongly suggests that she *had* trusted herself in her interaction with the physician.

The care Janet took in assessing the available evidence revealed not only that she was optimistic about being epistemically responsible, but also that she was making a considered attempt to act in that way. Because of the reflexive nature of self-trust, people who are self-trusting must take some responsibility for meeting the relevant commitments, rather than merely being optimistic in that regard. Mere optimism would suggest that they were assuming only the role of the truster, not of the trusted one as well. Janet clearly took both roles.

Furthermore, in taking responsibility, she was displaying a virtue that is social, which is true of moral integrity. Following Calhoun (1995), I stated in chapter 2 that integrity is a social virtue because it involves standing for something. In so standing, we take forward-looking responsibilities for ensuring that what we value is preserved or established. We also accept the backward-looking responsibility of being accountable when we fail to honor our commitments. We do that out of respect for ourselves or others, and in either case we fulfill social responsibilities. Moral responsibilities to the self have a social dimension, particularly in societies that depend on their members to be responsible for themselves to a large extent. Janet displayed concern for herself and her physician by aiming to be epistemically responsible, and thus she exhibited a social virtue: further evidence that she trusted herself.

After the physician doubted her, Janet's self-trust quickly turned into self-distrust. She became pessimistic about whether she had been responsible in encouraging him to believe that she was pregnant. She felt that way not only because her claim might not have been grounded in "real" evidence, but also because she might have been hysterical in making it. In other words, it might have been inconsistent with the evidence *she* valued.

The physician's insensitive remark, "You told me you were pregnant and I believed you" caused Janet's self-trust to disappear. The comment certainly does not reflect much compassion for Janet, who might have been seriously upset by the news that she was never pregnant. Especially if it turned out that was true—that she *had* never been pregnant—the physician's behavior made it unlikely that she would ever trust herself again in interactions with him (that is, if she ever did interact with him again). Such a barrier to her autonomy is profound and the physician would be obligated to try to remove it. His moral integrity would demand that he make amends to Janet in a way that allowed her to regain some self-trust.

The physician could have known that he had made that moral mistake by noticing Janet's guilt or shame and also by realizing how careful she and Richard had been in charting her cycle. He must have assumed, at least in the beginning, that they had been careful; why else would he have accepted her charts as evidence? Thus, signs that a patient trusted herself in a relationship with a physician are a concerted effort on her part to meet certain moral commitments and moral responses of guilt or shame when it appears that she failed to live up to them. At times those feelings may be warranted, such as when patients trust themselves too much; and in such cases, physicians may be justified in lowering the patients' self-trust. Yet even then they must act in ways that are respectful of the need patients have to trust themselves to some extent. The trick is to try to lower their self-trust without destroying it altogether.[4]

Expectation about What I Stand For

Continuing with the theme of self-trust as a nonprototypical variant of trust in others, we should consider whether one other feature of interpersonal trust was implicit in Janet's attitudes: the expectation that the one trusted has relevantly similar values to the one trusting. That feature is important because otherwise we could not assume that the one trusted is committed to doing what we trust that person to do. We do not trust her to have the relevant commitment simply by being optimistic about her moral integrity, because she could act on different moral commitments and still maintain her integrity. That would be the case if she were to interpret her moral responsibilities differently than we do. However, that worry does not arise with self-trust, does it? The issue of how my values might differ from those of the trusted person when I trust myself does not arise, for she and I are one and the same. Thus, it seems that we do trust ourselves to act on certain moral commitments simply by being optimistic about our moral integrity. Thus, Janet had only to be optimistic about her competence and moral integrity to have trusted herself in the domain of interaction with the physician.

Throughout, I have described Janet's self-trust as though it concerned her present behavior: she trusted herself to be telling the truth when she told the physician that she was pregnant. But what if her trust initially targeted her future behavior? For example, what if she trusted herself before ever meeting the physician or even before attempting to conceive that she would be epistemically responsible in such situations? Would the issue not then come up of whether she would continue throughout her interaction with the physician to hold those values of honesty or truthfulness? She might all of a sudden feel that it is more important to her just to assume that she is pregnant rather than be completely honest with herself and with the physician (however farfetched that might sound). Most self-trusting attitudes probably concern our future behavior, in which case we might have to expect that in the future we will be committed to the values we now hold that are relevant to our trust in ourselves.

But to have that expectation we would have to question our commitment to our present values, and that in itself would reveal that we are not committed to them. What if Janet were not as devoted to natural family planning as she seems to be? In fact, she suspects that if she were in a relationship with someone who was not as concerned about it as Richard she probably would not have been spent all that time taking her temperature. On hearing that, most of us would question Janet's commitment to natural family planning (which, in some moral systems would constitute a moral commitment). It seems to be just a fad for her or a need to be perceived as one who believes in that method. Moral values and preferences are distinct in that we can expect that our preferences for certain things (e.g., jogging) will not last long, whereas we cannot expect the same of our moral values.[5] The expectation that we will hold them in the future is implicit in our endorsement of them.

Thus, where Janet's self-trust was future oriented, her optimism that she would act with moral integrity or live up to the commitment to be honest about her pregnant state must have *implied* an expectation that her future self would be committed in that way as well. It would be redundant to add to a description of her attitude the expectation that her future values will line up with her present values.

Even though one might not expect one's values to change in the future, they might change nonetheless. When we modify our values for whatever reason, do we betray trust we might have had in ourselves to honor those values? That issue is complicated, especially since having integrity sometimes *requires* that we revise our commitments, rather than strive to meet those that are no longer appropriate, given new circumstances, new relationships, or new knowledge (Walker 1998; Babbitt 1996). If that is true, we do not betray our optimism that we will act with moral integrity when we change our values and act on new ones. But if we had trusted ourselves to act on our earlier values, it seems that we do betray ourselves. We betray the trust we had in our commitment to those values.

The best way to respond to that apparent paradox, I think, is to acknowledge that when we revise our values in ways that are compatible with maintaining our integrity and consequently we fail to meet our earlier commitments, we might cause some harm or disappointment to others, but we do not betray ourselves. If the relevant commitments were to others, we might disappoint them and even betray their trust. But if we no longer care about our earlier commitments, why would we betray ourselves by not living up to them? Consider a scenario in which Janet's commitment to natural family planning had been solid, but was then compromised. She had promised Richard that she was as committed as he was, but after the miscarriage, she decided to take the Pill. She could not possibly handle another pregnancy, not now anyway, and she wanted to feel as protected as possible from becoming pregnant. In the past, she would never have considered such a move, but now her fear of pregnancy was stronger than any fear that the Pill was unnatural. Since her priorities changed, it is not clear that Janet betrays herself by making that decision; however, she certainly might disappoint Richard.

We can conclude that the attitudes Janet described are profoundly similar to interpersonal trusting attitudes. She expressed optimism, then pessimism toward her own competence and moral integrity, and her optimistic attitude presupposed an expectation about the similarity between her current values and the values of the trusted person (i.e., her present or future self). Those attitudes are similar enough to interpersonal trust and distrust that we would call them self-trust and self-distrust, respectively. So now that we know that such attitudes are meaningful, how distinct are they really from other attitudes that are self-regarding? What about self-confidence and self-respect? Why identify self-trust as an important condition for autonomy when it might not be different from those other attitudes?

Self-Trust versus Other Forms of Self-Appreciation

To sort out ways in which self-trust is different from other forms of self-appreciation, let me introduce another case of miscarriage in which a woman expressed a number of different self-regarding attitudes in describing her experience. Sheila miscarried at eleven weeks' gestation in her second pregnancy. She wrote that at the first sign of trouble,

I knew immediately that I would lose the baby. It was the first moment after the full-term pregnancy and 11 weeks of the present pregnancy that I felt scared that something could go, and in fact now was going, wrong. The possibility of problems had never before occurred to me. I knew things could go wrong in pregnancy but I felt I was one of the lucky ones who would sail through it with very little alteration from the norm . . . I was totally shattered. I was someone whose life revolved around bodily activity. I had worked hard to gain control in body action, to be aware of how my body moved and reacted to stimuli. I was fit and healthy. Now I felt I had lost all control of my body. I kept bleeding and there was nothing I could do about it. It was the first feelings of guilt (feelings that were to remain with me for a long time)—that I of all people should be experiencing something other than a normal pregnancy. "Pregnancy is not an illness"; you should be able to continue as before with slight limitations. I, who enjoyed fitness and activity, was now faced with terrible guilt. Had I brought on this miscarriage myself? Oh, why had I been so selfish to go away the weekend before? I had felt the need for a break so had . . . gone to the mountains. I must have overstrained myself—it was my fault. If only . . . (Hey et al. 1996, 21)

In her complex reaction Sheila displayed attitudes that targeted three abilities she thought she possessed before the miscarriage: her ability to act responsibly in pregnancy, her ability to sail through pregnancy without experiencing problems, and her ability to control her body action.

Sheila's belief that she would be responsible in her pregnancy was an attitude of self-trust. The guilt she suffered after her miscarriage because she thought she had caused it by hiking in the mountains is evidence that she was committed to being responsible for the welfare of her potential future child. Further evidence comes from a decision she made to exert herself less than usual on the hike; earlier in her story she explained that she had taken it easy by slowing her pace and carrying less weight than usual. That decision was informed by her knowledge that "'Pregnancy is not an illness'; you should be able to continue as before with slight limitations." Thus, Sheila was optimistic that she was competent to act responsibly in her pregnancy, that she knew what that would take, and that she was committed in that regard. Her view of that commitment changed when she miscarried. She had been selfish to go on the trip, for she must have overstrained herself. Her self-trust was quickly replaced by distrust.

Sheila's guilt might seem unreasonable, especially to people who know that it is highly unlikely that hiking caused the miscarriage. However, it is important to interpret those feelings against the background of pronatalist norms that require women to go to extreme lengths to care for their children (or potential children) and that presume that it should be second nature for most women to know how to care for them.[6] Those norms imply that Sheila should have known how to protect her potential child and should have ensured it was protected. What she assumed was guilt might even have been shame in what she perceived to be her own shortcomings as a mother and as a woman.

Sheila's attitude toward her moral responsibilities in pregnancy was distinct from her attitude about sailing through it in one important respect. She was optimistic that she would be responsible, but she did not simply *expect* that would happen without conscious effort on her part. On the other hand, she merely expected to sail through, for as she said, "the possibility of problems had never before occurred to me." That attitude was one of self-confidence rather than self-trust. In being self-confident, "you do not consider alternatives" (Luhmann 1988, 97). Rather than appreciate the risk that you might disappoint yourself or others, you simply expect that you will act competently.[7] With self-trust, you appreciate the risk but you are committed to trying to avoid it.[8] Furthermore, if you fail to honor your trust, you respond with shame or guilt, whereas if you fail to do what you had been confident you would do, the expected emotional response is shock or surprise. Sheila was shocked when she discovered that her pregnancy was not running smoothly.

Sheila's self-confidence is understandable given the dominant messages that women receive about pregnancy in Western society. "The literature . . . , our mothers, and shared collective common sense make it seem that having a baby as the result of being pregnant is as automatically guaranteed as rain in June" (Hey et al. 1996, 127). In fact, miscarriages occur in over 50% of all conceptions,[9] a statistic that our society tends to ignore for a number of reasons.[10] Some of those reasons have to do with the cultural construction of femininity as a characteristic of childbearing women. For instance, that role is meant to be positive, yet to keep that meaning alive, it is important that women maintain a rosy picture of childbearing.

Such societal messages are probably what made Sheila unprepared for the possibility that she would miscarry. She was also unprepared to deal with what went on her body at that time. She had learned that by maintaining a high level of fitness she could control how her "body moved and reacted to stimuli." That control was lost with the miscarriage: "I kept bleeding and there was nothing I could do about it," "I had lost all control of my body." In those moments Sheila felt incredibly vulnerable, and she admitted in her story how dependent she was on others, including her partner, as a result.

I suspect that Sheila's attitude about her ability to control her body action was one of self-reliance. I doubt that it was self-trust, since it is hard to imagine what moral commitment she could have been living up to while striving to have such control. It is possible that she was self-confident about that ability, but it is more likely that she was self-reliant, given that her attitude was probably grounded in fear of losing control. Sheila seems to have what our society labels "the superwoman syndrome," which some women develop in response to societal pressure that they excel in their careers and at the same time take most of the responsibility at home for child care and domestic work (Hey et al. 1996, 140). Women who are overburdened with those responsibilities sometimes find that they can cope only if they can be optimistic about being in control over virtually every aspect of their lives. They live at least under the illusion of complete control. Sheila's desire to have control over her body seems to be a symptom of that so-called syndrome[11]; she probably feels that if she were to lose control in one area of her life, the rest of her life would fall apart.

Thus, Sheila's response to miscarriage was a mixture of diminished self-trust, diminished self-confidence, and diminished self-reliance. Her story illustrates well that the motivation we expect from ourselves with self-reliance is different from that with self-trust. The former does not presuppose anything about our moral character. Neither does self-confidence, but it is a more extreme emotion than either self-reliance or self-trust.

Self-confidence is not an attitude of optimism; it has a kind of certainty to it that is missing with self-trust and self-reliance.

What about self-respect? How does it differ from self-trust? One might assume there is little difference between the two because self-respect, like self-trust, concerns our moral character. However, only one type of self-respect actually involves the appraisal of our character—what Stephen Darwall (1995) called "appraisal self-respect"—whereas another type is about recognizing that we are beings with moral worth who deserve to be treated respectfully—what Darwall called "recognition self-respect." Appraisal self-respect overlaps significantly with self-trust. The former targets our moral character and the competencies we develop as a result of that character (Darwall 1995, 187).12 Thus, a woman could respect herself for having the moral integrity to become a capable mother, and she could also trust herself in that regard.

How does self-trust differ from appraisal self-respect? One clear difference is that we are vulnerable when we trust ourselves, but not when we appraise our character. Vulnerability is a key feature of self-trust, which I discuss in detail in the next chapter. Why do we incur vulnerability when trusting ourselves and not when respecting ourselves? The reason, it seems, is that with self-respect, we are optimistic that we possess moral integrity, whereas with self-trust, we are optimistic that we will act with integrity, not merely that we possess it. The focus on our actions entails a risk of disappointment or harm that is absent with appraisal self-respect. One might object that we sometimes say, "we have enough self-respect that we will display moral integrity," which seems to imply that appraisal self-respect *is* about whether we will act morally.13 I think that statement has to be filled out, however; the point is that we respect ourselves enough *to be optimistic* that we will act with moral integrity. In other words, we respect ourselves enough to trust ourselves in the situation at hand. Appraisal self-respect and self-trust do tend to reinforce one another,14 yet they are distinct.

Relationality of Self-Trust and Distrust: The Need for Uptake

Significant work has been done in feminist philosophy on the topic of self-respect to show how that attitude is socially constituted, in the sense of being developed and preserved only through supportive social relations (Dillon 1992, 1997; Meyers 1989). However, similar work does not exist about the relationality of self-trust and self-distrust. We have seen that those attitudes can be influenced by the reactions of others to our behavior (e.g., Janet's physician's comment about her claiming to be pregnant) and by societal norms, including oppressive norms (e.g., pronatalism). I want to end the chapter by discussing one domain surrounding miscarriage where women can feel profound self-distrust and where their attitudes are shaped significantly by the responses of others. The domain is of their emotions, or of their ability to understand and express their emotions clearly. When people are not sympathetic to how a woman feels about her miscarriage and fail to give uptake to her feelings, she can become distrustful of her competence and commitment to understand them well.

Consider the following case. Anna had a positive pregnancy test at six weeks' gestation, but the next day she started bleeding severely and miscarried. Subsequently, she suffered a lot of emotional confusion. She had a loving partner who was deeply concerned about what she was going through, but he did not seem to be able to help her. "I found it really difficult to express just how difficult I was finding it emotionally after the miscarriage, and . . . I guess partly because I didn't know anyone else who'd miscarried and I felt sort of like, well, it was only six weeks. It wasn't like I'd lost, . . . lost a baby or that I'd had a stillbirth or something like that, . . . and you know that maybe I shouldn't be as upset as I was" (Leaney and Silver 1995).

Often women and their partners are pressured not to grieve after miscarriage because people tend not to view the fetus's death as an event that warrants grief. That is reflected in their responses, where a common example is that it was a "blessing in disguise; the baby would have been deformed" (Hey et al. 1996, 129). Miscarriage is interpreted as a blessing not only when the fetus might have had an abnormality but also when the pregnancy was unwanted and the woman, or couple, was trying to decide whether to terminate it. It is a blessing that they did not have to make what might have been a very difficult decision. But even when women miscarry unwanted pregnancies, they and their partners can experience the event as a significant loss and be confused or even offended when others suggest that they should be relieved.[15] Whenever a woman feels incredible sadness about a miscarriage and others respond as if there is little to be upset about, she may become confused about her feelings and, in particular, about whether their intensity is warranted.

Immediately after miscarriage, grief and stress are common for women and tend to be more severe for them than for a male partner (Alderman et al. 1998). Moreover, the degree and duration of grief likely vary depending on the meaning the pregnancy had for the woman. Women value and define their pregnancies differently, and that influences how they respond emotionally to miscarriage (Layne 1990; Madden 1994). Cultural factors can come into play and so can such factors as class, race, and disability. Societal disapproval of reproduction among poor women, especially women of color[16] and those with disabilities can influence how positively they view their pregnancies. Anna's pregnancy had a positive meaning for her, which is why her grief was so intense.

However, when it came to understanding her grief Anna felt a kind of "emotional incompetency." She "found it really difficult to express just how difficult [she] was finding it emotionally after the miscarriage." There are two reasons why she might have felt that way. One is that she may have thought that most people would be unsympathetic to her feelings if she were to try to articulate them, and the other is that she was simply having trouble articulating them. She may have thought that people she knew, including her partner, could not be truly sympathetic, since none of them had ever experienced such an event (as far as she knew).[17] They might not be sympathetic because, "it was only six weeks," and "it wasn't like I'd lost . . . a baby." Anna may have been imagining people interpreting her miscarriage as relatively insignificant and that made her to try to interpret it that way as well.

Anna was confused about how she was feeling, however, and not just concerned that others would be unsympathetic. She was somewhat persuaded by the view that the death of her fetus did not warrant profound grief, although she experienced that level of grief nonetheless. That must have made her confused about whether her feelings were warranted, and maybe even uncertain about whether they were caused by the fetus's death. She might have been thinking that if its death was insignificant, it could not have triggered those feelings. They must have been caused by something else, in which case they were not feelings of grief over the death of a fetus. They could have been feelings of anger over how others treated her (perhaps she assumed that they blamed her), or about an imagined death of an imaginary entity that had greater moral or personal significance than her fetus. Of course, they also could have been caused by abrupt hormonal changes.

The two reasons Anna found it difficult to express her feelings might be interconnected. She might have been confused about her feelings and about the occasion that triggered them *because* of the lack, or presumed lack, of sympathy from others. One theory of feelings explains why that may have been the case (1997). According to Sue Campbell, until others give "uptake" to our feelings, that is, until they recognize them as the same sorts of feelings as we do, we often cannot be certain what they are feelings of (1997). If I assume that I am angry but people around me keep saying that I am bitter, I am probably going to be uncertain about what I really am feeling. Feelings are individuated (their content is defined) collaboratively through their expression (Campbell 1997). Their individuation is determined both by how the person with those feelings interprets the occasion that triggered them, and how the people to whom she expresses those feelings interpret that occasion. If people do not see how the occasion warrants the kinds of feelings she claims to have, she will probably be confused about what those feelings are about (Campbell 1997, 109, 110).

This theory is helpful in understanding the difficulty that some women have in sorting out their feelings about miscarriage when those feelings clash with the way society expects them to react emotionally. Their emotional turmoil is no coincidence if people do not acknowledge their feelings or even deliberately try to discourage them out of an interest in perpetuating our society's rosy view of childbearing. Using Campbell's account, we can explain the emotional confusion brought on by such comments as "it was a blessing in disguise" or "it could have been worse: you could have lost a baby." Women who have miscarried need listeners who will give uptake to their feelings, rather than demand different feelings. Those are people who have some idea of the degrees of emotional significance that miscarriage can have for women.[18]

We can refer to Anna's competence in understanding her feelings, and whether she trusts or distrust it, even though it is dependent on the uptake of others. We can assume about that competency that it is relational in the sense that one's ability to exercise it depends on whether one has opportunities to collaborate with sympathetic others. The competency can manifest itself only if those opportunities exist.

Anna distrusted her emotional competence in the context of miscarriage, and that distrust was profoundly relational because of how it was shaped by common societal reactions. The moral commitment she endeavored to live up to while attempting to display some emotional competence was the commitment to express her emotions clearly and to act appropriately given their content. She struggled to express her emotions, which means that she wanted her behavior to communicate them; that is, to be suitable behavior given what her emotions were. And she probably wanted to do that not only for her own sake, but also for the sake of her partner and for others to whom she felt some obligation to be reasonably clear about her feelings. She was striving to meet that moral commitment, but was pessimistic that she was competent to live up to it.

Anna's case, perhaps more than the others we have explored, illustrates how relational attitudes of self-trust and self-distrust can be. Other people and the norms of society can have a profound effect on whether we can trust ourselves. By recognizing that fact moreover we can fully appreciate how health care providers can be morally obligated to respect patient self-trust as part of their duty to respect patient autonomy. Health care providers in these examples had a responsibility to ensure that they did not cause or perpetuate the women's distrust in themselves.

Conclusion

Self-trust is a relational attitude distinct from other attitudes that are self-regarding, and it is coherent despite the interpersonal nature of our trust prototype. Together with self-distrust, it is also highly relevant to women's experiences of pregnancy and miscarriage. Like Janet, many pregnant women feel trust or distrust toward their ability to know what is happening in their bodies. Like Sheila, they either trust or distrust their competency and commitment to be morally responsible in pregnancy. If they miscarry and blame themselves for it, which is not uncommon among women (James and Kristiansen 1995), their distrust in that domain may be severe. Some women might even have trouble trusting themselves again to be responsible for a potential future child. Finally, if women miscarry and are barraged with comments such as "it was only six weeks" or "you could just try again right away," chances are many of them will experience distrust at the level of their emotions, as Anna did.

Self-distrust is not always morally problematic, however, and neither is self-trust always unproblematic. Say that a woman is overly optimistic about her ability to know her own body in pregnancy, which might have been true of Janet, even though it turned out that she was right about being pregnant. Especially if she had relied solely on her embodied awareness of pregnancy, Janet might not have been justified in trusting herself as much as she did. If that were true, she would have made herself vulnerable to serious disappointment and perhaps even to a lowering of her self-respect. As I mentioned in the previous chapter, some bioethicists discuss how vulnerable patients tend to be when they trust their health care providers because of their own limited medical knowledge. Next I hold that patients can be vulnerable to the same degree when they trust themselves, and especially if they trust themselves too much or too little.

4

Vulnerability with Self-Trust Compared with Interpersonal Trust

Some people seem to be able to trust themselves well throughout a variety of domains. When they face difficult life choices they can usually trust that what they will decide to do is right for them and that they will live up to whatever commitment they make to follow through with their decisions. These are not people who are arrogant necessarily or overly confident. They are people who know themselves well, know what they have to do to be happy or comfortable in their lives and what they are capable of achieving. Although they also must have knowledge of the external world that allows them to identify what it is that makes them happy or comfortable, self-knowledge is probably the main factor in their justified optimism toward themselves. A woman with such optimism who makes a considered decision to continue a pregnancy can proceed with little fear or anxiety about how she will cope with the outcome. Her self-knowledge allows her to trust herself without becoming seriously vulnerable. Overall, she is probably less vulnerable in trusting herself than she is in trusting other people.

It is reasonable to ask, though, to what extent that ability is a mark of privilege of being raised in a social environment where she learned to appreciate herself and her talents (a privilege that is not necessarily coexistent with the absence of oppression). How is such biographical information relevant to the degree of vulnerability that any of us incur in trusting ourselves? One might think it is not relevant, that our social circumstances are not an issue here. What is at issue is our ability to introspect our own needs and desires, to reflect rationally on our past successes or failures and to compare them with our present situation. People who can do that can trust themselves well (i.e., in a justified way) and whether they can do that is a matter of how rational and intelligent they are.

One might argue that regardless of our social environment, we are less vulnerable in trusting ourselves than in trusting others. Trudy Govier hesitantly endorsed that view: "With self-trust, the predictability of success [i.e., of our trust being honored] or failure may be greater: we should know better what is going on because it is, after all, our own self that we are trusting. That is not to say, obviously, that our self-knowledge is perfect. Risk remains: we are vulnerable to our own failings" (1998, 95). I contend that how vulnerable we are to our own failings with self-trust depends considerably on the nature of our social environment. And I explain how acknowledging that fact should lead us to suspect that we can be as vulnerable in trusting ourselves as we are in trusting others. That point is relevant to assessing the value of patient self-trust: its value diminishes the more vulnerable the patient is to harm by trusting herself. Also relevant is the relation between self-trust and autonomy, because if we were not terribly vulnerable to getting things wrong with self-trust, our self-trust would promote our autonomy most of the time. (Self-trust that is unjustified inhibits our autonomy, as I argue in chapter 6.) The barrier to autonomy of too much self-trust would not be as significant if we were not as vulnerable in trusting ourselves as we are in trusting others.

Comparing the degree of vulnerability with self-trust and interpersonal trust is not merely an epistemic issue, however. It is important to ask not only how vulnerable we are to failure, but what are we vulnerable to or what are we putting ourselves at risk for? I refer to the last as the moral dimension of vulnerability with self-trust and interpersonal trust, and believe that the two are symmetrical in that dimension. In other words, the harms to which we are vulnerable in trusting ourselves are the same as the potential harms with interpersonal trust. And I contend that one is particularly susceptible to those harms in either case if one is abused or oppressed.

Vulnerability as a Prototypical Feature of Trust

In the Introduction I wrote that it is important to be able to trust others and to trust oneself in situations of vulnerability.[1] However, we also usually incur vulnerability *by* trusting because the trusted one might not honor our trust.[2] Trust and vulnerability are so closely intertwined in our minds that vulnerability to unfulfilled trust must be prototypical. In previous chapters I modeled trust on a prototype theory of concepts and maintained that self-trust is nonprototypical because it is self-regarding. Still, it shares most of the prototypical features of interpersonal trust, to which we can now add vulnerability.

Vulnerability is prototypical because of the moral nature of trust. The morality of trusting attitudes extends both to the motivation of the trusted person and to that person's competence. We want people we trust to act with moral integrity in promoting our interests (or the interests of others) and to have the moral competence to know what that takes. If they exhibit both, their actions will truly be aimed at furthering our good, which is what we want in trust relations, according to Baier (1995). In my theory, what we want from people we trust in prototypical relations is that they further certain aspects of our good in certain domains; rarely do we place our entire well-being in the hands of another. Still, Baier's discussion about promoting the good of another is relevant to my theory. She explains that the task is rarely mechanical and therefore that people we trust must use their judgment rather than act with "mindless regularity." "Turning over to automatic pilot is not often a serious possibility for those whose goal is the good of another—or even when their goal is their own good" (Baier 1995, 136–137).

Take the example of a reproductive endocrinologist who gives all of her new infertility patients the same (dry) speech about infertility, taking little time to consider how a woman or couple is coping with the information or how relevant that information is to them. The endocrinologist is not expressing the kind of concern that would warrant patients trusting her, and neither is she displaying the moral competence necessary to perform the task of disclosure. She probably will not succeed in conveying all of the information that is relevant to her patients because of differences in their informational needs, arising from differences in their concerns about infertility and in their cognitive capacities. To be competent to do what trust demands of her, she has to use her judgment, because what trust demands is furthering at least some aspect of the good of another.

Even when attending to patients' physical needs, physicians have to use their judgment. They must be mindful of what is going on with each patient because, "[w]hen all is said and done, [they] cannot anticipate every contingency even in a disease [they] understand well" (Pellegrino 1991, 74). Going on automatic pilot as a physician usually guarantees incompetence. Trustworthy physicians do not lapse into that state (or they do so only rarely) because they are committed to the welfare of their patients. They feel compelled to use their judgment for moral reasons, not simply because they want to be good at the art of medicine or because they want to avoid malpractice suits.

If furthering someone's good requires using one's judgment, people we trust must have what Baier called "discretionary powers." They must be able to use their discretion in deciding how best to serve our interests. And since it makes us vulnerable to allow them to do that, vulnerability must be a prototypical feature of trust. As soon as we try to remove that feature by controlling the behavior of others, we cease to trust them. We are no longer optimistic about their moral integrity, as we are giving them no room to express it. We do the same thing to ourselves when we try to eliminate every possibility that we will mess up and fail to fulfill our trust in ourselves. A pregnant woman can read every book, article, and magazine she can get her hands on about how to act appropriately in pregnancy; but she does not trust herself to do what is appropriate if she never allows herself to use her own judgment in that regard. Of course, the mere act of checking her judgment against that of experts does not undermine her self-trust (Baier 1995, 139, 140). Moreover, it is probably a rational thing for her to do. However, for her to be self-trusting and to live up to that trust, she has to apply the information she reads to her own life and do what is right for her and for her fetus given available resources and whatever responsibilities she has to others.

Thus, being optimistic that someone is competent and committed to furthering our good involves granting that person some discretionary power, which in turn makes us vulnerable as the trusting person. Because of the moral dimension of trust, vulnerability is a key feature of trust relations and of self-trust. Note also how that is consistent with the connection between vulnerability with trust and potential betrayal; we tend to think of trust as something that engenders vulnerability because it can be betrayed. Feeling betrayed is a moral response to the failure of another to act out of moral concern for us. We are vulnerable in being optimistic about someone's moral integrity because the person might abuse the discretion we grant him and consequently, betray our interests.

Self-Trust and Vulnerability: The Moral Dimension

One might wonder whether we could ever betray ourselves. Is self-betrayal a coherent concept? The answer is relevant to whether we are vulnerable to the same sorts of harms in trusting ourselves as we are in trusting others. Trust can be either betrayed or disappointed, and the potential harms of betrayal are greater than the harms of disappointment. Betrayal can engender or perpetuate low self-respect and damage our ability to trust ourselves and others in the future. I claim that betrayal is possible with self-trust, and that it can occur for many of the same reasons as it does with interpersonal trust.

Betrayal versus Disappointment

Baier (1995) wrote about the different ways that other people can fail to live up to our trust: "[s]ometimes, like Elizabeth I of England, we have to report that we 'in trust have found treason,' or, less regally, betrayal, or, even less pompously, plain let-down" (130). From that quotation one might assume that betrayal and let-down are distinct categories for Baier; but, in fact, they differ only in degree. In her taxonomy, betrayal is more severe than let-down, although both occur because someone fails to live up to a commitment to us out of some moral failing, such as weakness of will or deception. By contrast, I will refer almost exclusively to such failure as betrayal, although I sympathize with Baier's suggestion that the word is too harsh to describe some moral failures, and I identify one area in which let-down occurs.

According to Baier, whenever one is merely disappointed, one did not really trust in the first place. "We all depend on one another's psychology in countless ways, but this is not yet to trust them. The trusting can be betrayed, or at least let down, and not just disappointed. Kant's neighbors who counted on his regular habits as a clock for their own less automatically regular ones might be disappointed with him if he slept in one day, but not let down by him, let alone had their trust betrayed" (Baier 1995, 99). In Baier's view, whereas being disappointed is appropriate when someone fails to do what one relied on him to do (as Kant's neighbors relied on his regimented habits), being more than disappointed is appropriate when one relied on another's goodwill. However, in my view, trust is not about someone's goodwill; it is about moral integrity. And once we accept that fact, we can begin to understand why it is sometimes disappointed. People can fail to live up to our trust because their circumstances prevent them from acting with moral integrity or because integrity requires that, in response to changes to their circumstances, they revise their moral commitments. In either case, they disappoint our trust, but they do not necessarily betray it.

We can believe that someone has betrayed our trust, but be wrong; we can feel betrayed but not *be* betrayed. Feelings of betrayal often surface when people we trust have to revise their moral commitments and forego doing what we trusted them to do. Take Maria, who is a patient at a prenatal clinic and who trusts her primary obstetrician, Dr. Morales, to perform a procedure he scheduled and that she needs at that particular time in her pregnancy. Dr. Morales is unexpectedly detained and cannot be present at Maria's appointment, even though he had said that he would be. As a result, Maria might feel betrayed by Dr. Morales, even though she may not have *been* betrayed. If Dr. Morales's integrity demanded that he place his commitment to another patient above his commitment to Maria, and furthermore, if he is accountable for the distress he caused Maria, he acted with moral integrity. In chapter 2, following Walker, I interpreted integrity as being reliably accountable for our actions. In her words, it is "reliability not only *ab initio,* but also *post facto,* in various reparative responses, something including changes of moral course" (1997, 73). Dr. Morales did not betray Maria's trust if he was reliably accountable in a moral way, for that is how we expect people we trust to act. If Maria, alternatively, expected Dr. Morales to act *immorally* by putting his commitment to her before his commitments to any other patients, no matter what unforeseen circumstances arose, she did not trust Dr. Morales. She simply relied on him to act out of some intense devotion to her as his favorite patient perhaps, or out of some threat she made to him.

What if Dr. Morales cannot repair damage to his relationship with Maria? Sometimes when the circumstances of the trusted person stand in the way of his honoring our trust, he cannot be accountable for failing to honor it. Say that the procedure Dr. Morales missed was amniocentesis, and a physician Maria had never met performed the procedure. Amniocentesis can be difficult psychologically not only because it carries a risk of miscarriage (approximately 0.5%), but also because of what it entails. A large needle is inserted into the woman's womb to extract amniotic fluid while ultrasound monitors the position of the fetus to keep the needle a safe distance away. The woman can look at the screen to see what is going on—the needle piercing the womb, the fetus's body near by. If she earlier pictured her womb as a safe place for her fetus, she may lose that perception, at least temporarily. If she felt a kind of integrity to her pregnant body, she may lose that feeling. Especially if the person performing the procedure is someone she does not trust completely, she may continue to feel long afterward that her bodily integrity has been compromised.[3]

If Maria felt compromised specifically by having the procedure performed by someone other than Dr. Morales, Dr. Morales may not be able to make amends to her. He might try by explaining why he had to miss the appointment and apologizing, but Maria might feel betrayed nonetheless. Whether she actually was betrayed, however, would depend on how reasonable (or unreasonable) she is being in blaming Dr. Morales and in refusing to accept his apology. Maria alone does not determine whether Dr. Morales was accountable for failing to meet his commitment, for accountability is an objective notion. Making amends is subjective (you make amends if the other person feels that you have). Consider an abusive man who continually makes amends for his behavior by persuading his partner that it will never happen again (even though it has happened many times before and he has not taken steps to try to avoid it, e.g., by seeking counseling). The abused woman might let him off the hook every time, even though he was never really accountable for his actions. Being accountable is what defines integrity, not making amends.

It is clear that the abusive partner—the trusted person—lacks moral integrity, although in other cases, it is not so clear. Sometimes, there is confusion about what the trusted person has to do to salvage or maintain her integrity, and about whether we should relieve her guilt or shame for failing to meet her commitments. Drawing a sharp line between when trust is betrayed and when it is disappointed is often difficult in practice.[4] It may even be impossible in some circumstances.

One situation that is probably neither betrayal nor disappointment but simply let-down is when we cultivate trust in those who have shown little evidence of integrity in the past, and who once again fail to act with integrity. Most philosophers who have written on trust agree that trust cannot be willed, but it can be cultivated (Baier 1995; Holton 1994; Jones 1996; Govier 1998, 170–174). We cultivate trust by narrowing our attention to what little evidence exists for a person's trustworthiness. The task involves, in other words, "a selective focus of attention toward the grounds for trust and away from the grounds for distrust" (Jones 1996, 16). Those grounds, in my trust theory, include whether the person has the capacity for moral integrity, whether he is competent in the relevant domain, whether he shares certain moral values with us, and how he perceives the nature of our relationship. I might cultivate trust in someone based on little evidence that he holds the values that I want to be able to trust him to have (because I am his parent, say, and I want him to acquire those values). Alternatively, I might know that the other person holds relevant values, but also know that he suffers acutely from weakness of will. In that case, if he does not honor my trust, he fails to act with moral integrity.[5] However, given that I had little evidence that he would *ever* honor my trust, it seems inappropriate to say he betrays it, or that I am justified in feeling betrayed. On the other hand, disappointment would be inappropriate, as that would suggest I was only hopeful rather than optimistic about his trustworthiness. If I truly trusted him, I would react more strongly than that. Thus, when we cultivate trust in someone but that person fails to act with moral integrity, we are let down. Betrayal is too harsh and disappointment too mild for such circumstances.

To summarize, betrayal or let-down occurs when people we trust do not act with moral integrity, whereas those who disappoint our trust maintain their integrity but do not do what we trusted them to do. Such conceptual distinctions are relevant to self-trust as well as to interpersonal trust. With the former, we are vulnerable to changes in our circumstances that require us to reorder or reevaluate our commitments, and act on different commitments than those we had trusted ourselves to meet. However, we are not vulnerable to betrayal in such cases, unlike with interpersonal trust. There, if we act on different commitments than those which others trusted us to meet, we betray their trust if we are not fully accountable for our actions. But in chapter 3 I stated that we do not betray trust in ourselves when we revise our values in ways that are compatible with maintaining integrity. If we no longer care about our earlier values, in no reasonable sense do we betray ourselves. On the issue of when betrayal can occur, self-trust and interpersonal trust are therefore asymmetrical; yet in other respects in which one can fail to be trustworthy, they appear symmetrical. For example, I could cultivate trust in myself in a domain in which I know that I am highly susceptible to temptation, and if I fail to honor my trust it seems reasonable that I would be let down.

As with interpersonal trust, making practical distinctions between betrayed self-trust and disappointed self-trust may be difficult. When my circumstances change and I revise my commitments, sometimes I am uncertain about whether the revision is truly justified and whether I should let myself off the hook for harm I cause by denying my earlier commitments. Especially if the harm is significant and borne largely by me, I might feel that I have betrayed myself, even though, perhaps, at most I should feel disappointment. Consider a woman who was always committed to the pro-life movement but finds herself in an unwanted pregnancy and decides that her only choice, given her circumstances, is to have an abortion. Racked with guilt later on, she might feel that she has betrayed her moral commitments, but only because she has now forgotten how desperate she was. In light of her circumstances then and her current moral commitments, disappointment is the only justified response.

Notice how I referred to betraying one's moral commitments, which might seem more coherent than "betraying oneself." Beyond saying that "self-betrayal" sounds odd, it is hard to know why worry over whether we could betray ourselves exists. Perhaps it is because of the close association between betrayal and deception. The classic way to betray others is to deceive them about what one's moral commitments are, about whether one intends to act with moral integrity, or about how competent one is.

With self-trust and betrayal, the issue arises from a philosophical perspective of whether self-deception is a real phenomenon. Philosophers
have long noted that it seems paradoxical for someone to play the role of
deceiver (believing X) and that of the deceived (believing not-X) simultaneously. However, the most persuasive theorists in that debate are surely
those who demonstrate how self-deception is possible, where the most
common explanation is to posit different levels of consciousness or different subsystems of the mind, the contents of which can conflict.[6] Self-
deception is so common in the lives of many that it must be real, and thus
it must be possible to betray ourselves.

Self-betrayal can also occur because of weakness of will or insensitivity. I might trust myself to care for the needs of another, but when it
comes time to fulfill those needs, I am too weak-willed or too insensitive
to attend to them properly. In either case, self-deception would not enter
into the picture if I had been intending all along to live up to my trust
and never tried to kid myself about whether I had the opportunity to do
so. In other words, I never tried to deceive myself into thinking that I
could not possibly have acted on the relevant moral commitments because of changes in my circumstances.

In the end, whether being weak-willed, insensitive, or self-deceiving
can lead to self-betrayal or betrayal of one's commitments is immaterial
to a discussion of whether we are vulnerable to the same harms with self-
trust as we are with interpersonal trust: we are, because we can at least
betray our commitments. I now argue that the harms of the betrayal of
self-trust or interpersonal trust are more severe than with trust that is
merely disappointed. And people who are abused or oppressed are more
susceptible than others to those harms.

Harms with Betrayal and Vulnerability with Abuse and Oppression
When trust is betrayed or disappointed, we experience whatever harm
comes from its not being fulfilled. Returning to Maria and Dr. Morales,
whether Dr. Morales disappoints or betrays Maria's trust is irrelevant to
whether Maria actually feels the harm of having her bodily integrity compromised. Nonetheless, betrayal often brings with it additional harms,
such as diminished self-respect, diminished capacity to trust oneself and
others, and diminished autonomy. The idea that harm comes through

having a reduced capacity to trust or a heightened capacity to distrust implies that one is vulnerable in distrusting as well as in trusting.

One of the harms that can accompany the betrayal of self or of others is loss of self-respect. This can happen when we are betrayed, because betrayal implies that we are not worthy of respect. It can negatively affect what Darwall (1995) called "recognition self-respect"; that is, the respect we have in acknowledging ourselves as beings with inherent moral worth who deserve to be treated respectfully by others. Our recognition self-respect is endangered when we betray ourselves as well as when others betray us. If in betraying ourselves we fail to live up to a serious moral commitment, we might feel unworthy of others' basic moral consideration. More commonly, self-betrayal damages our "appraisal self-respect," our respect for our own moral character (Darwall 1995), which is called into question by our failure to act with moral integrity.

Usually, the more serious the betrayal, the more serious its impact is on our self-respect. Citing the work of Cathy Roberts on women and rape (1989), Susan Brison (1997, 30) wrote, "[v]ictims of rape and other forms of torture often report drastically altered senses of self-worth, resulting from their degrading treatment. That even a single person—one's assailant—has treated one as worthless can, at least temporarily, undo an entire lifetime of self-esteem." Such treatment betrays whatever trust one has in the world to be a safe place, a place where one can trust people to treat one with at least minimal respect. And if that trust is betrayed in a way that is profoundly degrading, as Brison suggests, the loss of self-worth or self-respect can be severe.

Feelings of betrayal can also interfere with our ability to trust, especially if the betrayal is severe, such as that which stems from violence. Being betrayed by others can cause us to doubt our ability to trust others well or at least damage that ability. If rape, for example, shatters the survivor's sense of the world as a safe place, she will no longer know when trust or distrust is appropriate. Those who suffer abuse in childhood may never develop the ability to trust or distrust well, and they are at serious risk of further abuse without those skills. As Judith Herman (1992, 111) explained, "[t]he risk of rape, sexual harassment, or battering, though high for all women, is approximately doubled for survivors of childhood sexual abuse" (Russell 1986).

Abuse can also lower or inhibit self-trust. Trudy Govier (1993b) re-ferred to a small study by Doris Brothers (1982) showing that the great-est problems with trust caused by incest and rape lie in the survivor's trust in herself. Brison's work on trauma and the self is helpful in inter-preting that finding. Survivors of rape and other forms of violence often suffer from posttraumatic stress disorder, some symptoms of which are heightened startle response, flashbacks, and hypervigilance. Those symp-toms "render involuntary many responses that were once under volun-tary control" (Brison 1997, 27). With traumatic memories flooding back at unexpected moments and with abnormally heightened responses to startling events, the survivor is no longer predictable to herself. Hence, she can no longer trust herself as she once did.

An inverse relation probably exists between abuse and self-trust, such that heightened abuse brings about lower levels of self-trust. That causal sequence is particularly relevant to some women in pregnancy, as women who are abused tend to experience increased abuse in pregnancy (Stew-art and Cecutti 1993). If their self-trust subsequently decreases, so will their reproductive autonomy, assuming that self-trust is necessary for autonomy.

Self-distrust, like self-trust, makes one vulnerable. When it is pervasive it prevents us from forming and acting on autonomous beliefs and desires. It also perpetuates low appraisal self-respect, for people who do not trust themselves to test their moral character never learn to respect it. Low self-respect, in turn, can prompt mental illness, particularly depression.

Different mechanisms of psychological oppression can encourage the harms of too much self-distrust. Abuse that causes psychological harm is a form of psychological oppression if "it is directed at members of a group simply because they are members of that group" (Young 1990, 62). Oppression is something that happens only to groups. Thus, if a woman is a target of abuse because she is a woman (the abuse stems from hatred of women or from an unconscious or conscious belief that women deserve to be subordinated in that way) the abuse is an instance of sex-ist oppression. That is true especially if it incorporates certain modes of psychological oppression, such as objectification or stereotyping (Bartky 1990). When oppressive stereotypes or oppressive forms of objectifica-tion become embodied in the subject, they breed self-distrust.[7] People who think of themselves as objects, for example, have difficulty trusting themselves to do what objects cannot do (e.g., advocate for themselves, have beliefs and desires of their own).

Distrust that is interpersonal also carries with it potential harms that may result, ultimately, from oppression. Some of that harm is interpersonal, for when distrust is ill-deserved or even when it is well-deserved, and its source is discrimination or a reaction to being discriminated against, it stands in the way of a potentially rewarding relationship. Distrust that is ill-deserved can also harm the distrusted individual, for if distrust is an attitude of pessimism about someone's moral integrity, it must be a sign of disrespect for that person. Conversely, trust is a sign of respect. We do not trust people merely for instrumental reasons, contrary to the view of many social contract theorists for whom trust is just another mechanism, like a contract, for furthering our self-interest. (I discuss that view in more detail in the next chapter.) Trust has instrumental value surely, but it is also a moral attitude that we extend toward people we respect.

To illustrate the potential harms of interpersonal distrust that is motivated by oppression, consider the situation in South Carolina around testing pregnant women for substance use. The Medical University of South Carolina instituted a policy in 1989 that allowed for nonconsensual drug testing of pregnant women and arrest and incarceration of those who tested positive (Roberts 1997, 164–176). Of the forty-two women arrested under that policy, all but one was black (the one white woman arrested had a black partner, as a nurse judiciously noted in her chart). The assumption that those numbers reflect proactive and racist policing is warranted, given that a study reported in the *New England Journal of Medicine* found that those who commit so-called prenatal crimes are *not* disproportionately black; in fact, substance use in pregnancy is slightly more common among white women (Chasnoff et al. 1990). The unfair targeting of black women for prenatal drug testing is potentially very harmful. It is disrespectful of the commitment of these women to the well-being of their children, and it discourages those who are pregnant and use drugs from seeking prenatal care. It stands in the way of their developing any beneficial relationship with a prenatal care provider.[8]

When oppressive norms encourage distrust or the betrayal of trust, it certainly harms those with less power; however, it can also harm those with power over others. As I suggested, the latter may suffer the interpersonal harm of foregoing relationships that are potentially edifying because of distrust. And if they betray others, they can be harmed together with the betrayed, particularly if they own up to what they have done. In that case, the consequences for both parties may be similar: diminished self-respect, diminished self-trust (e.g., in one's ability to live up to one's moral commitments, in the case of the betrayer) and, ultimately, diminished autonomy. Such harms may even befall abusers, although the harms they suffer hardly compare with those they inflict.

The harms for abusers may be short-lived, particularly for those who are members of privileged groups, because of how privilege often allows one to make amends relatively easily. Whether one can make amends (as opposed to whether one is accountable) determines the level of harm one suffers in failing to meet one's commitments. Harm, which is subjective, is minimized as long as the trusted person is made to feel that he has been accountable (i.e., as long as he is able to make amends). People with privilege can more easily make amends than those who are underprivileged because privilege affords one credibility.[9] We tend to hold the integrity of those who are privileged to great heights, but assume paradoxically that if they falter, it was simply a mistake on their part or it was beyond their control. For example, the man who abuses his children is often described as subject to uncontrollable violent impulses, whereas the woman who does so is depraved and unnatural. The white health care provider who distrusts that the black pregnant patient is drug free simply because she is black is victim of the mistaken view that black people tend to abuse harmful substances more often than whites, and, perhaps, that black women tend to make bad mothers.[10] But since the media tend to foster both of those impressions, how is the white provider really to blame (or so the reasoning would go)? On other hand, if a black patient displays distrust toward a white health care provider who individually does not deserve such treatment, the patient is ungrateful at best and paranoid at worst.

People who are privileged tend to recover quickly not only when they have betrayed someone but also when they themselves have been betrayed.

One might think that people in power have more to lose from betrayal, since they have the power to lose. The king who is betrayed by his not-so-loyal subjects may no longer be king. But kings, or those who might be kings, have a remarkable way of bouncing back when things go wrong (as long as they do not lose their heads in the process). They usually appear on the political scene in the near future, often stronger than they were before. Still, their renewed strength is often due more to patronage than to resilience or dire struggle.

Thus, people who are oppressed, compared with those with privilege, are especially vulnerable to the harms of trusting or distrusting badly in part because if they are implicated in those harms, it is more difficult for them to make amends. I argued that point while insisting simultaneously that the potential harms of trusting badly are the same whether trust is self-directed or other-directed. In either case, one is vulnerable to disappointed trust and to betrayed trust, where the potential harms of betrayal or perceived betrayal are greater. When betrayal itself is exceedingly cruel, as with incest or rape, it can cause extraordinary damage to the survivor's perception of herself and of her social world.

Trust and Vulnerability: The Epistemic Dimension

One might accept that with self-trust we are vulnerable in the same ways that we are with interpersonal trust, but object that we are never *as* vulnerable as we are in interpersonal trust relations. In other words, one might agree with Govier (1998) that with self-trust, "we should know better what is going on because it is, after all, our own self that we are trusting." She assumes that we are better knowers of ourself than of others and therefore we are less vulnerable to getting things wrong with self-trust. Whether either of those statements is correct, however, depends considerably on the nature of our social environment. Only those with supportive social environments can reach their full potential for self-knowledge, which is greater than their potential for knowing others. In that context a "supportive" social environment is one where we receive honest and respectful feedback about what our selves are like.

The traditional reasons for believing Govier's claims about self-knowledge are dubious. Some philosophers have thought that introspection was an infallible or nearly infallible route to self-knowledge. And since it is not a route we can take in understanding the mental attitudes of others, and we do not have an equally clear and accessible route to understanding them, presumably we are in a better position to know ourselves. However, we have good reason to doubt the perspicacity of introspection. It alone cannot ground claims to self-knowledge for it does not allow us to detect certain psychological and physiological conditions, prevalent throughout the population, that promote self-misunderstandings (Kornblith 1998, 55). Examples are paranoid personality disorder, color blindness, and even being emotionally well-adjusted, which tends to involve "a degree of optimism [that] can, on no reasonable construal, be justified by the facts" (Kornblith 1998, 58).[11] Such conditions can occur in mild or severe forms (thereby causing mild or severe degrees of self-misunderstanding), and they can distort not only our introspection, but also our external perception of ourselves, which is an alternative route to self-knowledge.

No matter how weak our powers of introspection may be, however, it still might be right that with self-trust "we should know better what is going on" (Govier 1998). Kornblith is skeptical of our ability to know ourselves well, but he does not think that self-knowledge is impossible, and he does not rule out the possibility that we know ourselves better than others. We can know that we do not suffer from such conditions as severe paranoia if we are "experiencing no difficulties at work or . . . have good relationships with others" (Kornblith 1998, 59). Since we are in a better position to gather such evidence about ourselves than about others, we should be in a better position to know ourselves well than to know others. Notice that the evidence Kornblith identifies as being relevant to our self-understanding does not come from introspection alone or from our perception of our behavior. Rather, it comes from outside of ourselves. To know ourselves well, we rely on feedback from others about what our selves are like. And how good their feedback is influences how much we can know about "what it's like to be [us]."

That view of self-knowledge as a social phenomenon coincides with the feminist view of the self as inherently social. Persons are essentially "second persons," to use an often-quoted phrase from (Baier 1985). They are "heirs to other persons who formed and cared for them" (Baier 1985, 85, quoted in Brison 1997, 14) who determine in profound ways what it is like *to be* them. Persons are social or relational beings not only because other persons shape who they become, but also because others give meaning to their experiences and to their feelings (as we saw in chapter 3 in discussing the need for uptake; Brison 1997, 14; Scheman 1983). Brison supported that claim when she explained that people who have been traumatized need others to bear witness to their horror so that they can truly come to grips with what happened to them. They cannot assuage the guilt they feel by finally accepting that they themselves did not cause the rape or torture, feelings that are "practically universal" among trauma victims (Herman 1992, 53), unless others lead them on that path to self-knowledge.

People who continually experience abuse are often in a very bad position to obtain self-knowledge. It is obviously a barrier to have someone constantly insinuate or just say outright that one is inferior, that one is worthless, that one is just asking for it. For many people who are abused, that is their only feedback because abusers typically strive to isolate their victims and prevent them from seeking aid or emotional support from others, thus making the psychological domination complete (Herman 1992, 79, 80).

On the other hand, people who are oppressed usually have mixed sources of feedback that either improve or worsen their ability to gain self-knowledge. People who live in communities that are made up of members of their same social group (e.g., black or First Nations communities), or who establish collectives of people who are socially situated in similar ways (e.g., women's collectives) often receive very positive feedback. Whereas in the wider culture oppressive stereotypes prevail, within those communities or collectives the challenge to those stereotypes can be great.

However, not everyone from a minority group has liberated communities from which to draw strength. People in such communities are also not immune to outside social influences. Furthermore, relatively new community members can carry around the baggage of oppressive stereotypes about who is incompetent and who lacks integrity. One barrier to knowing oneself and to trusting oneself well (to which I have only alluded) is distortion of our prototype for trust by oppressive stereotypes. Privilege bestows credibility precisely because of the oppressive nature of our trust prototype. Overall, the prototype of the trustworthy individual in Western society is male, white, straight, and, perhaps most important, professional.

A person who fits that description and has all the mannerisms, style of speech, and dress that we normally associate with professionals is immediately accorded respect (Young 1990), and is therefore trusted immediately by many of us. Unless such a person has already shown himself to be untrustworthy, it is rare that people would react to him with suspicion or with the general sense that he should prove his competency or integrity (unlike, e.g., with women in male-dominated professions).

The influence of oppressive norms about who is trustworthy and who is not can make one as susceptible to getting things wrong with self-trust and self-distrust as one is with interpersonal trust relations, no matter where one is located socially. Oppressive trust prototypes often encourage people who are oppressed to distrust themselves where self-trust is warranted,[12] and to trust others who neither have their best interests at heart nor the knowledge to be able to say with authority what their best interests are. But notice how those prototypes can also interfere with whether or not people of privilege get things right in trusting themselves or others. To assume that you alone are trustworthy in a group of people who are inferior to you in the social hierarchy is often to trust yourself too much. And to assume that people who are inferior should immediately be distrusted is often to make a grave error. You can be as wrong about yourself as you are about others—whether you are high up or low down on the social totem pole—particularly if feedback reinforces oppressive assumptions about who should be trusted.

Hence, it is not obvious that most of us are more likely to get things wrong with interpersonal trust or distrust than we are with self-trust or self-distrust. That is because the dominant trust prototype in our culture reinforces stereotypes that can lead us astray in trusting ourselves or others, whether or not we occupy subordinate social positions. People who are oppressed are generally more susceptible to *harm* from getting things wrong than people of privilege, but they are not clearly more susceptible to getting things wrong.

Conclusion

Let us return to the example of the person who just seems to be able to trust herself well. She must have a supportive social environment because otherwise she would not have the requisite self-knowledge. Furthermore, the support she receives cannot be unconditional in the sense that she is told that whatever she does is right or good, which is something that a person of privilege might be told as a condition of privilege. A supportive environment for good self-trusting and self-distrusting is one in which people receive truthful and constructive feedback about themselves and learn to have a trust prototype that is nonoppressive. Wherever one is situated socially, if one inhabits such an environment for a considerable length of time, one will probably become a good self-truster and self-distruster.

One will also probably be better at trusting oneself than at trusting others. Being in a better position to gather evidence about how one's own life is going, as opposed to how other people's lives are going, is an advantage if the evidence is reliable. But if an oppressive prototype for trust distorts one's perception of the evidence or influences the evidence, the advantage is lost. One can be equally vulnerable, therefore, in an epistemic sense in trusting oneself as one is in trusting others. And in a moral sense one can be vulnerable to the same degree of harm.

One harm of betrayal of trust that I mentioned is loss of autonomy, which is a consequence of trusting oneself less in response to being betrayed. The way that oppression and abuse can interfere with getting things right with self-trust and with self-distrust has serious consequences for autonomy. Getting things right is important, in my view, because too much self-trust is a barrier to autonomy just as too little is. Thus, to understand the relationship between self-trust and autonomy fully, we have to understand what it means to get things right. We need a theory, in other words, of the justification of self-trusting attitudes.

5

Feminist Politics and the Epistemology of Trust

I have shown how oppression can be a barrier to getting things right with self-trust and interpersonal trust. But how does it influence whether we are justified in adopting these attitudes in the first place? Surely, the political dynamics of our culture influence whether we actually do trust ourselves and others in various domains. For example, a woman may not trust herself to engage well intellectually with a man if the general sense in her culture is that women are intellectually inferior to men. A gay man who has not yet dared to venture from the closet may not trust his straight friends to understand his sexual orientation. Especially if clear evidence points against such distrust—by any objective measure, the woman is as intelligent as her male counterpart; the straight friends are strong proponents of gay rights—we would question whether such attitudes are rational or justified. Yet many of us could understand why they might be justified given the social context, which is sexist and homophobic. In light of that context, the attitudes may not seem unreasonable at all. How, then, are we to evaluate trusting and distrusting attitudes in a political climate of oppression? I answer that question using a social and reliabilist epistemology of trust and distrust that makes the justification of those attitudes relative to the sociopolitical position of the subject.[1] I use that epistemology in later chapters to explain what it means to say that justified self-trust is important for patient autonomy, and what health care providers can do to try to bolster or preserve it.

Some philosophers have noted the relevance of sociopolitical positioning to an epistemology of trust (Webb 1992; Scheman 2001; Jones 1996, 21), yet they have done little theorizing on that topic. In her paper that began the surge of interest by philosophers in trust, Annette Baier (1995, 127) wrote, "[i]f the network of relationships is systematically unjust or systematically coercive, then it may be that one's status within that network will make it unwise of one to entrust anything to those persons whose interests, given their status, are systematically opposed to one's own." She implied that it would be irrational to trust and perhaps even rational to distrust in such circumstances; however, she did not offer a theory to support her intuitions. Other ethicists followed suit, showing reluctance to theorize about the rational justification of trust and distrust. That reluctance stems most likely from the opinion that "trust and distrust are not entirely, or even mainly, rational matters. We do not always trust and distrust on the basis of a careful consideration of the relevant evidence . . . " (Govier 1993a, 156). It may be neither rational nor irrational for the woman to distrust her judgment in the face of sexist norms or for the gay man to distrust his friends; it may simply be non-rational.

Whether "careful consideration of the relevant evidence" is even necessary, though, before it could be rational to trust or distrust is debatable, particularly if we are talking about *epistemic* rationality. Something is rational in an epistemic sense as long as it is likely to be true, whereas something is rational in merely a strategic or instrumental sense if it is likely to fulfill a particular desire (de Sousa 1987, 163–165). Most moral philosophers would agree that trust is never purely instrumental; it always has a moral element that precludes us from trusting others merely for our own benefit. Rather, we trust in hope that the trusted one will display moral integrity. Thus, if trust and distrust are at all rational matters, their rationality must be understood epistemically,[2] at least to some degree. We want it to be true that the trusted person has moral integrity as well as the competence to do what we trust him to do. An important difference between the two models of rationality is that whereas theories of strategic rationality recommend decision procedures or strategies for rationally adopting the relevant attitude, theories of epistemic rationality do not always offer decision guides. Nor do I in the epistemology of trust that I defend. Trust or distrust can be rational without our having carefully sifted through relevant evidence, evaluating it in terms of set rules for rational decision making, and even without being aware of what that evidence is. Stricter epistemic demands would be unreasonable, I contend, particularly for conditions of oppression, where forces that undermine our ability to trust some people can be so subtle that they are beyond conscious detection.

Before exploring alternative epistemic demands for rational trusting, however, we need some sense of what kinds of mental attitudes trust and distrust are. Are they beliefs about someone's trustworthiness? Are they emotions? The answer influences what we can say about their justification: "[I]f a theorist analyzes trust as (perhaps among other things) a belief . . . then that theorist has committed herself to saying that trust is justified only if the one who trusts is justified in forming the belief constitutive of trust" (Jones 1996, 5). It may not be possible for the woman who distrusts herself or for the gay man who distrusts his friends to be rationally justified if distrust were a belief about someone's untrustworthiness. These people are distrusting in the face of some contrary evidence as I implied, and we are usually not justified in forming beliefs in such circumstances.[3]

Trusting Emotions and Their Paradigm Scenarios

Think of someone in your life whom you trust. For me, it is my physician, Sue. I have always trusted Sue to give me good advice about my health and to be sincere in her concern for my well-being. I trusted her from the first time I met her because of her friendly smile and because good friends of mine recommended her as a family physician. I believe that Sue is trustworthy, but is that the best way to characterize my attitude toward her, to call it a belief? No. Further exploration into the nature of that attitude will reveal that it resembles an emotion, but not a belief, and an emotion that has particular perceptual and behavioral components. In trusting people, our attention is drawn toward features of their behavior that tend to confirm their trustworthiness, and we exhibit trusting patterns of behavior.

The idea that trust is an emotion that carries with it distinct patterns of attention was developed by Karen Jones (1996, 11–14), who drew on an influential account of emotions as ways of seeing the world (de Sousa 1987; Calhoun 1984; Rorty 1980). I propose that a model of emotions as behavioral attitudes can also help us to understand why trust is an emotion. I expand on Jones's account in that respect, and also by discussing how we come to have emotions according to a theory of emotions we both rely on: that of Ronald de Sousa. Interpreting trust in light of de Sousa's theory allows us to presume that trust is learned through association with "paradigm scenarios," which are profoundly similar in structure to prototypes (see chapter 2). Furthermore, like prototypes, they can be politicized, which is relevant to a feminist epistemology of trust.

To say that emotions involve perceptual and behavioral patterns of response is simply to say the following.[4] When we have a particular emotion—fear, let us say—we are attuned to information that grounds our fear, and we tend to ignore or deny information that would discount it (in that sense, our emotion is "informationally encapsulated"; de Sousa 1987, 152, 195). We also exhibit behavior that people would normally associate with someone who is scared. So if what we fear is a snake that briefly crossed our path, we would not easily be convinced that the reptile had slithered away or that it never actually posed a threat to us. We are also physically tense, staring down at the ground no doubt, with a look of fear on our face.

Behavioral responses are key elements, for they often allow us to identify whether someone is having a particular emotion and what the object of that emotion is (Campbell 1997, 77). When our only evidence for someone's emotional state is her behavior, we have to understand the typical patterns of behavior for different emotions to know what kind of state she is in. Furthermore, to know what her feelings target—that is, what their objects are—we must study her behavior closely. Emotions are not purely subjective in the theories I describe (de Sousa 1987, 143): they represent emotive properties of objects in the world or of states of affairs (i.e., properties of those objects or states that tend to elicit certain emotions in a given culture). To evaluate how well our emotions do that, we have to determine what they represent, which often requires that we know their distinctive patterns of behavior. Take trust. When someone is clearly trusting but will not admit it—say that person is in a vulnerable position but is unexpectedly calm—we must be able to understand from that person's behavior exactly *who* she is trusting.

To be able to evaluate trust in terms of its epistemic rationality or irrationality, the attitude must be not merely representational, but also cognitive (in the sense that it involves some kind of appraisal of one's situation).[5] If the perceptual element of emotions, as described by de Sousa, Calhoun, and Rorty, were entirely noncognitive, modeling trust on such a theory would be unwise in a chapter on the epistemology of trust. The perceptual model is cognitive, although not in the traditional sense of being propositional, a point Calhoun (1984) makes most clear.[6] She stated that emotional perception is guided by distinctive "cognitive sets"[7] or "interpretive frameworks" that lack a propositional structure. Those sets furthermore explain why such perception tends to be limited to certain "fields of evidence" (Jones 1996, 11).

Limits of that sort reveal that emotions are "not primarily beliefs, although they do tend to give rise to beliefs," such as beliefs in someone's trustworthiness (Jones 1996, 11). Emotions are more informationally encapsulated than beliefs, meaning that they do not change as easily in response to contrary evidence. Of course, that is not to say that emotions are not responsive to evidence at all. To return to our snake, we could be convinced at some point that it had slithered away, and consequently our fear would subside.

So why would I model my trust in Sue, my physician, on the perceptual and behavioral accounts of emotions I have outlined? Consider what would happen if a rumor was milling about that Sue was negligent in caring for one of her patients. If I really trusted her, I would find it hard to believe the rumor, would I not? Trust has specific patterns of attention because someone genuinely trusting is resistant to counter-evidence (Jones 1996, 11, 12; Baker 1987, 3). And that is true of someone who is self-trusting as well as someone who trusts others. When people are not easily swayed by the opinions of those who might question their abilities, we tend to think of them as self-trusting (Govier 1993b).

Trust and distrust are also characterized by certain behavioral patterns, as the following illustrates. I claim to trust Sue, but all the while I am finding out as much as I can about her credentials as a physician. Also, at my appointments with her, I peer over her shoulder when she writes in my chart. Back home, I telephone her frequently, trying to find out the results of tests she has performed, even though she told me that she would call as soon as the results came in. Clearly, we would question whether I really trust Sue because my behavior is inconsistent with the behavioral patterns we normally associate with trust. One might say that what my behavior reveals about the focus of my attention is what makes it incompatible with trust; I am acting as though I am ever watchful for and anticipating evidence of untrustworthiness. So my attitude is characterized ultimately (and entirely) by my perceptual patterns, or so the objection goes. To respond, it is my behavior that signals those patterns in the first place. The behavioral evidence is not irrelevant, for without it we could not identify where my attention is focused. We could not conclude that, in fact, I am *dis*trusting Sue.

In supposedly enlightened cultures where sexism, racism, and other forms of oppression persist often in subtle ways, we commonly use behavioral patterns to identify and evaluate trusting attitudes. The white guy who claims that he is not racist but who moves to the other side of the street when a black man walks toward him *is* suspicious of black men, probably because of racist stereotypes about their integrity. A woman who says that she trusts herself to be confident and assertive with men to whom she is sexually attracted, but who shies away from them entirely, in fact probably does not trust herself. The reason may lie in bitter tension between her desire to be assertive and the training she has received to be submissive and accommodating with men.

Still, that woman might say that she trusts herself because she is trying to cultivate self-trust in a domain where she showed little evidence of trustworthiness in the past. Although it is not possible to will oneself to trust, as philosophers have insisted (Jones 1996, 15; Holton 1994), it is possible to cultivate trust in someone who is not obviously trustworthy. The usual method, as I noted in chapter 4, is to strive to keep one's attention on whatever small amount of evidence exists for the person's trustworthiness.[8] Thus, the woman who wants to be more assertive could continually remind herself of a relationship she once had with a man in which she did assert herself at times. She could also avoid spending time with people who are likely to undermine her confidence in that domain and seek out those who are more likely to bolster it. Using those strategies, she could trust herself even if the preponderance of evidence points against her trustworthiness. Such cases illustrate why trust is probably not a belief in someone's trustworthiness. Although it is likely that the situation I describe is not amenable to the formation of a belief,[9] it is compatible with the formation of a trusting attitude.

A further point, which establishes that trust is not constituted entirely by a belief, is that one can have the belief without having the trusting attitude. I might believe that someone is trustworthy but I have never actually trusted her, or even considered trusting her, because she tends to operate in domains with which my life does not intersect. Consider Jan, a pediatrician. I have committed myself to a life without having children of my own, but because reliable sources tell me that Jan is a great pediatrician, I believe that she is trustworthy. However, since I have never had to trust her for anything (we are not even friends),[10] my belief does not amount to a trusting attitude. The belief and the attitude are separate.

Thus, we can conclude that trust and distrust are not beliefs, but emotional attitudes with perceptual, behavioral, and cognitive dimensions. To say they are not beliefs does not rule out that sometimes they are grounded in beliefs or give rise to them. If a time came when I needed a pediatrician, having changed my mind about having children, I would probably call on Jan. The trust I would have in her then would be founded on my belief in her trustworthiness. Trusting attitudes need not have such a foundation, however; the case of the woman cultivating self-trust is an example.

Knowing that trust and distrust fit the model of emotions as perceptual and behavioral attitudes allows us to begin to understand their justification and how it might be influenced by oppressive norms. A further claim of one proponent of the perceptual model, de Sousa (1987), is that emotions are learned through association with paradigm scenarios. These are clear cases in which it is appropriate to have the relevant emotion; and they involve a "situation type," which identifies the characteristic objects of the emotion, and a set of normal responses to that type of situation (de Sousa 1987, 182). Take envy. A common paradigm scenario is feeling envious when someone else receives an award that you coveted. The situation type is the other person getting the reward and the normal response is envy, with all of its characteristic patterns of attention and behavior. The ability to associate that response with a scenario that is clearly mediated by culture must be learned (which does not deny, of course, that our capacity for envy might be rooted somewhat in our biology).

How do paradigm scenarios compare with prototypes that structure our concepts, according to prototype theory? Perhaps, learning prototypes for different emotions teaches us only how to use emotion concepts: in other words, how to recognize situations that warrant or exemplify different emotions. On the other hand, paradigm scenarios give us the know-how not only to categorize emotions, but also to respond appropriately to relevant situation types. They are prescriptive, in other words, as well as descriptive. But apparently prototypes have "just such a dual character: they encode information about the world in a way that combines procedures of categorization with decisions about actions" (May et al. 1996, 7; Flanagan 1996, 25).

Prototypes and paradigm scenarios may also differ in that prototypes are artificial exemplars—they combine salient features of many real exemplars—whereas paradigm scenarios are real exemplars. The one I gave for envy is entirely recognizable; it does not have the features of many different scenarios crammed into one complicated one. Nonetheless, paradigm scenarios could become complicated in that way. They can be "revised in the light of competing paradigms that are applicable to the situation at hand" (de Sousa 1987, 187). Through revision they could become as artificial as prototypes.

To see how that process might go, take a situation that somewhat resembles the paradigm scenario for envy, but is also similar to a common one for pride. I am a parent with a child who is successful in many areas in which I had always hoped to shine. I have to figure out what mixture of emotions is appropriate in such circumstances. I have to modify my habitual responses so that the attitude I adopt accurately represents the situation. I should probably also then refine my scenarios, especially those for envy, to account for situations in which the target of my emotion is my own child. Knowing when to refine our paradigm scenarios and when to modify our habitual responses is a skill in itself; and it is an important one for knowing how to have emotions that reliably depict their objects (i.e., emotions that are justified).

Sometimes people have to have the opportunity to experience new paradigm scenarios. People raised in oppressive social environments are usually taught oppressive paradigms for different emotions. For example, many women learn that situation types that warrant shame are those in which they are sexually abused by men, or alternatively, in which they experience intense sexual pleasure. To end exist oppression, women must be liberated from such scenarios.

Paradigm scenarios for trust are not immune from influence by oppressive norms and stereotypes (see also chapter 4). That people from dominant social groups are habitually trusted whereas people from outside of those groups are not reveals that our concept of trust is structured in terms of paradigm cases and that the paradigms tend to mirror social divisions along the lines of race, gender, class, and so on. In dominant Western culture, the paradigm of the trustworthy individual is a white, straight, middle-class man, and people who are situated apart from that ideal are "not normally taken at their word" (Webb 1992). "A woman says she was raped; a young black man says he was beaten by the police; a lesbian says she was harassed at her workplace; none of them is accorded the immediate trust usually accorded to straight white men" (Webb 1992, 390).

Thus, trust and distrust are learned through paradigm scenarios, which themselves can be oppressive. We develop trusting attitudes by comparing and contrasting paradigm scenarios with the world, and hence, their justification must have to do with how well we do that. Because of the oppressive nature of the paradigms, part of that task will often be to modify our habitual responses to free them of such distortion. Now we need a theory to accommodate these insights. Let us consider first whether help is forthcoming from philosophers who have written about trust.

Reluctance to Theorize: Moral Philosophers on the Epistemology of Trust

When it comes to evaluating trusting attitudes, a fairly clear divide exists between moral philosophers and many political philosophers who embrace social contract theory. What I called above reluctance to theorize among ethicists is an extreme reaction, I think, to the way that many social contract theorists talk about trust and rationality. The latter assume that trust should be evaluated in terms of how well it maximizes the self-interest of the trusting person, and that wise trusting comes only through calculating the relevant person's trustworthiness. If you do not have clear and ample evidence that the person will do what you trust her to do, you really should not trust her in the first place. Moral theorists generally deplore that view, rightly I think, because of how it instrumentalizes trust and ignores how much of our trusting is unreflective, even unconscious, as well as grounded in a multitude of factors that defy calculation. Hence, someone such as Govier concludes that trust is not primarily a rational matter. I consider that trust can be rational epistemically even where no rational calculating is going on.

Russell Hardin (1996) exemplified the stance that many ethicists vehemently oppose. He implied that trust is justified only if constraints are imposed on trusted ones that require them to honor one's trust. The kind of evidence relevant to whether people are trustworthy, for Hardin, is the presence of external constraints. Either social devices are in place to ensure the cooperation of those people, or we know that they have fabricated constraints of their own to motivate them to live up to their commitments. I might "set my alarm clock on the dresser a few feet from my bed where I will have to stand to stop it noise," knowing that once I get out of bed, I will not return to sleep (Hardin 1996, 30). Having laid that trap, I can trust myself. And since my trust is grounded in reliable evidence, it must be justified.

Hardin's views about trust and its empirical warrant are questionable on a number of fronts. For one, it is not even clear that he is talking about trust, which arguably has a moral dimension (although he rejects that view). I can trust myself to get out of bed in the morning only if I am optimistic about my moral character and how it (not some external device) will motivate me to get up and face the day.[11] Self-trust is an attitude of optimism about one's own competence and moral integrity in a particular domain. Although at times it develops consciously with explicit evidence to back it up, usually it is unconscious and the evidence vague or dispersed throughout our lives so that we could not possibly do the kinds of calculations that Hardin prescribes. Complex factors go into our trusting attitudes, including many past experiences we cannot now recall and, with interpersonal trust, our general impression of the other person, which is not necessarily gained from a definitive set of qualities about that person.

The question of when to trust? is more complicated than most contractarian theorists would have us believe. The presence or absence of external constraints is not enough, particularly if trust is a moral attitude. Usually, the evidence we have of the moral character of others is scanty, and when it comes to our own moral character, we are vulnerable to self-deception. To aim for a set of rules for good trusting is to underestimate the problem. "There are no . . . useful rules to tell us when to trust or even when we should have trusted" (Baier 1995, 151).

Nor are there useful rules to tell us when someone else should trust himself or others. Especially when the other person is in a different social position than we are and therefore tends to receive different social feedback, it is often presumptuous of us to think that we know whether that person is justified in self-trusting or in trusting others. A central claim of this book is that when patients are unjustified in trusting or distrusting themselves, health care providers should try to lower or bolster their self-trust, respectively, in an effort to promote their autonomy. This chapter reveals the need for caution in applying that principle. Health care providers, and physicians in particular, are not always well situated to assess whether the self-trust or self-distrust of patients is unjustified. And there are no useful rules to offer them for overcoming the epistemic limits of their social position. (Although, as I suggest below, they might improve their understanding of how the conditions for good self-trusting and self-distrusting differ for people from different social groups by understanding more about what it is like to be members of those groups.)

Rather than offering rules for when trust is justified, most ethicists simply list factors relevant to its justification. In other words, they identify common "justifiers," which refer to the "facts or states of affairs that determine the justificational status of a belief [or attitude]" (Goldman 1999, 274). Lists by Jones, Govier, and Baier include such factors as the domain in which we trust the person and the social role that person occupies. Social role can be relevant even to whether one should trust oneself; for example, a physician might legitimately assume she is untrustworthy in a particular domain (e.g., social work) because the domain extends beyond her role in her profession.

Another common justifier is the political climate or political structure of our society (Jones 1996, 20; Baier 1995, 105; Govier 1998, 137–138), where to many of us, what is important about that structure is how we are positioned within it. For example, in sexist societies, women are so positioned as to be under the continual threat of rape or sexual assault. Learning to trust and distrust well in that kind of climate involves taking the threat seriously when trusting others. Ideally, their paradigm scenarios for trust become nuanced in response to it, and as a result, they are cautious about trusting men, particularly in situations in which they are most vulnerable to attack.

Political climate can also be relevant to self-trust. Whether I feel that I can trust myself as a middle-class white woman to understand what it is like to live as a poor black woman may depend on whether the dominant culture is classist and racist. If it is, structures will be in place to maintain my privilege that may largely be hidden from my view. If that is the case, I should not trust myself to make responsible claims to knowledge about the lives of people subordinated by those structures, given where I am socially located in relation to them.

The lists continue of justifiers for trust and distrust in trust theories by ethicists (especially Goviers 1993a), but justifiers are not incorporated into a theory of justification. The worry, perhaps, is that given how numerous those factors are and how varied their interactions can be, it is unreasonable to generalize about when to trust or distrust. Consider what that presumes, however, about justification. It implies that the epistemic subject has to be potentially aware of all justifiers and how they might combine to be justified in trusting or distrusting. Such epistemic demands are made only in internalist theories of justification. Internalists require that we be able to explain why our belief or attitude is justified for it to be justified. Many social contract theorists are among such epistemologists when it comes to the rational justification of trust and distrust (that is, insofar as the rationality of those attitudes for them is epistemic).

Internalist demands for the justification of trust and distrust are unreasonable for two reasons. First, to be able to heed them, it would be necessary to have constraints on what count as justifiers; if the number were unlimited, we would never be able to produce the required explanation (Goldman 1999, 274). To introduce such constraints is unreasonable because of how much of our experience goes into our trusting and distrusting attitudes. Second, to require that we know why our trust or distrust is justified ignores that oppressive influences on these attitudes are often so subtle or "mystified" (Bartky 1990) that they are beyond the reflective access of oppressed people. Only by mystifying forces of oppression can societies where people are supposedly "born free and equal" get away with oppressing groups of people indefinitely. Internalist demands on trust and distrust might even exemplify the kinds of epistemic norms that disenfranchise members of oppressed groups (Scheman 1993). They are unreasonable for them, given their social positions. Although more has to be said on that point, I raise it as a red flag against a feminist, internalist epistemology of trust and distrust. It, together with the other objection I raised, should persuade us to take a different road than social contract theorists in searching for a theory of when trust and distrust are justified. Instead, we should head toward externalism. Where justification is external to us, we are not required to understand why our attitudes are justified.

Jones (1996) hinted that trust lends itself to an externalist interpretation, particularly a reliabilist one. Reliabilism (of the kind I endorse here) says that our beliefs or attitudes are justified if they are formed and sustained by processes that tend to produce accurate representations of the world (Goldman 1992, 113). What matters to their justification is how they are generated, where the processes responsible for that can be largely unconscious. Jones supported a reliabilist theory by including what she called an "agent-specific" criterion in her list of justifiers, a criterion that establishes whether we ourselves are good "affective instruments"—that is, whether we tend to be good at trusting or distrusting in the relevant domain. If we are not:

. . . we should distrust our trust, or distrust our distrust, and demand a correspondingly higher amount of evidence before we let ourselves trust or distrust in the kinds of cases in question. Consider responses to physicians. We can imagine someone with a tendency to find authoritative and avuncular physicians trustworthy and physicians who acknowledge the tentativeness of their diagnoses and the limits of their art untrustworthy. Given how sexism shapes what we take to be signs of competence, we should be wary of our tendency to trust when an etiology of that trust tells us it is as likely to be caused by mannerisms of privilege as by marks of untrustworthiness. (Jones 1996, 21)

Assuming that sexism embeds cognitive error, trust-forming processes that are informed by it are unreliable. Agents who trust based on sexist assumptions of who is trustworthy are not reliable trusters. And they are unjustified in trusting the way that they do whether they realize it or not, which is something that Jones did not acknowledge. People might try to investigate whether they are "good affective instruments" by questioning the social norms that guide their trusting and distrusting attitudes (as in Jones's example). Alternatively, they can reflect on their past successes in trusting people who deserved to be trusted or in distrusting those who were untrustworthy. But whether they do or can perform such investigations is irrelevant to whether their trust is justified (if externalism about trust is warranted). For Jones not to acknowledge that fact reveals that she may be on the "internalist highway" herself, together with many social contract theorists.

Baier gives even stronger hints about the need to adopt an externalist theory of trust and distrust. She offered "a test for the moral decency of a trust relationship," which says that the continuation of the relationship "need not rely on successful threats held over the trusted or on her successful cover-up of breaches of trust" (1995, 123). Trust is "morally rotten" if it is generated through lies or threats, according to Baier, and also if knowledge of that fact by either party would "destabilize" the relationship. That is an externalist account of moral rottenness, for it focuses on the causal basis for our trusting attitudes. However, it is not clear that Baier meant it to be an account of rational justification. She often associated rationality with rule following, and at the same time acknowledged that no hard and fast rules are available for determining whether trust is morally decent. In other words, we can evaluate trust for its moral decency, but probably not for whether it is rational, as then we would require some "useful rules to tell us when to trust."[12]

I think we should take hints from Baier and Jones as instructive (despite the ambiguity that surrounds them) and accept that trust is a reliabilist concept. Modeling our theory after Baier's test for moral decency, we can say that trust is rationally justified when it is sustained not by deception, but by processes that are reliable in targeting persons who are competent and morally committed to do what we trust them to do. Such a theory requires elaboration, however, since other people—including those outside the trust relationship or external to the self-trusting person—can exert a positive, not only negative, influence on whether our trusting attitudes are justified. The reliable processes for the formation of those attitudes are inevitably social, I believe, which means that we must have reliable social feedback for whether we should be trusting for our trust to be justified. In extending the sources of feedback beyond the trusted person who might deceive us, I solve a worry that Baier had with her own test. She was concerned that it "ignores the *network* of trust" and how "any person's attitude to another in any given trust relationship is constrained by all the other trust and distrust relationships in which she is involved" (Baier 1995, 126). Epistemic agents *are* so constrained because of the social dimensions to the epistemology of trust and distrust.

A Feminist Social Theory of the Justification of Trust and Distrust

With reliabilism that is social, it often matters where we are positioned along familiar lines of gender, race, class, and the like in sorting out whether our trust or distrust is justified. Before determining why that is the case, however, we should decide whether to accept a social epistemology of trust. Justification is social where "the individual cannot make the needed connection between the evidence and the conclusion without relying, at least partly, on assumptions that the individual has not and perhaps cannot test for her- or himself" (Campbell 1998, 66). For example, my trust in Sue, the excellent physician, was grounded, initially at least, in the testimony of friends and hence it could have been justified initially only in a social fashion. If the justification of trust and distrust merely involved comparing and contrasting paradigm scenarios with the world, where such tasks were purely individual, we would not have a social epistemology. I propose that we need such an epistemology and the reason has to do with the social dimensions to our self-knowledge. To be reliable in trusting or distrusting ourselves well, we require some self-knowledge or must know that we are not self-deceived about our competence and moral integrity. Similarly, in trusting others, we rely on our knowledge of our ability to assess the trustworthiness of others, knowledge gained from past successes or failures in making such assessments. Since knowing ourselves and knowing that we are not self-deceived are both social processes, justification of trust and distrust must be social.

Self-deception is a potential source of distortion when trusting ourselves and others. How we come to deceive ourselves is revealing, furthermore, of the social nature of self-deception. What we do is place ourselves "where patterns of salience are likely to deflect attention away from what we do not wish to see" (Rorty 1994, 218). We are motivated by such a strategy, although usually not on a conscious level.[13] Whether we could even *be* motivated consciously is called into question by what philosophers deem to be the paradox of self-deception: being the deceiver (believing that X) and the deceived (believing not-X) simultaneously. Where self-deception is unconscious, evidence of it lies in our behavior and in inconsistencies between it and what we consciously believe or intend to do. Take Rhonda, who is self-deceived about her sexuality. Although she claims to be straight, her behavior clearly suggests otherwise (she is turned on by women and not by men, she is constantly flirting with lesbians, etc.). Only if she were to admit possibly to being a lesbian would Rhonda merely be confused about her sexuality rather than deceived about it.

We learn of self-deception when other people respond to inconsistencies between our behavior and what we claim to believe or desire. Their reactions tell us that we are self-deceived, although sometimes they prevent us from noticing the self-deception. For example, Rhonda's homophobic friend might be aware of how her behavior contradicts her proclaimed heterosexuality, but never challenge her to account for that. The friend might even go farther and actively reinforce her self-conception as heterosexual. Either possibility illustrates the point that self-deception is a "co-operative process"; "it works through sustaining social support" (Rorty 1994, 214, 215).[14]

We can be mistaken about our competence and moral integrity or about our ability to assess the competence and integrity of others not because we are self-deceived, but because we lack self-knowledge. As with self-deception, how we come to know ourselves reveals the social nature of self-knowledge. Drawing on the work of Kornblith (1998), I stated in chapter 4 that we come to know ourselves not only through introspection or from external perception of ourselves, but by responding to social feedback about what our selves are like. How reliable the feedback is determines how well we can know ourselves.

Given the social elements to self-knowledge and self-deception, reliable processes that generate justified attitudes of trust and distrust must be social, not merely psychological. We require reliable social feedback about how well we compare our paradigm scenarios for trust with the world.[15] Furthermore, our social position matters to whether our trusting attitudes are justified because often it determines how reliable our feedback is. I take as a form of distrust where gendered feedback is relevant to its justification the distrust that a woman can have toward herself in pregnancy.

Consider Eve, who distrusts her ability to make sound moral judgments about her prenatal care. Whenever the obstetrician seeks her informed choice for any aspect of her care (such as an ultrasound, antibiotics for a bacterial infection, or the mode of her delivery), Eve feels that any decision she would make would probably be bad for both herself and her fetus. Her self-distrust is manifested mostly in the continual demands she makes of the obstetrician to tell her what he would do in her circumstances. Whenever he answers that question, she defers to his judgment. She does not even contemplate whether that judgment is consistent with how she conceives of her responsibilities in pregnancy, since she does not trust her own judgment about what those responsibilities are.

Let me sketch the boundaries of where Eve's self-distrust would be justified or not, and also where it would be well grounded or not, meaning accurate in targeting her level of competency and moral commitment in using her judgment. Processes that produce justified trusting and distrusting attitudes are reliable but not foolproof, and hence, it is possible for those attitudes to be justified yet not well grounded. In terms of the justification of Eve's self-distrust, I also leave open the possibility that it falls inside of the boundaries of justification as an attitude that is only partially justified or partially unjustified. Trust- and distrust-forming processes can be reliable only to a partial extent[16]; that is, where they tend to produce accurate representations of people as trustworthy or untrustworthy only some of the time, or if they only somewhat resemble processes that are deemed reliable without qualification. They can also be reliable only in certain domains. Let us say that the domain relevant to Eve's self-distrust is one in which she is required to make potentially difficult moral decisions about her welfare and that of others close to her.

Consider first the boundaries determining where Eve's self-distrust is unjustified—that is, where the processes that produced it are unreliable. Of course, she would be unjustified if she has not engaged in the kinds of processes that would tend to give her well-grounded attitudes of self-distrust. For example, if she has not considered the social feedback relevant to those attitudes,[17] she would be unjustified. If that were the case, it would preclude her neither from being highly competent in making serious moral judgments, nor from being highly incompetent in that respect. What it would mean simply is that she is not always a reliable self-distruster in that domain.

Alternatively, the epistemic processes Eve engages in could be unreliable because the social feedback she receives reinforces mistaken attitudes of self-distrust. Thus, she responds to the relevant feedback, but it is unreliable. And the reason may be that people in Eve's community (including Eve herself, perhaps) have learned sexist paradigm scenarios for trust and distrust. The communal paradigms make it appropriate for women, let us say, to distrust their ability to make sound moral decisions, and hence appropriate for them to defer to the judgment of others (namely, men). In other words, the paradigms reflect a common social stereotype about women's incompetence relative to men in making serious moral judgments.[18]

Given that a sexist community may actually have deprived Eve of the ability to reason competently in a moral way, it is possible for her self-distrust to be unjustified (because feedback is unreliable) and at the same time, well grounded (an accurate representation of Eve's (in)competence). Eve may never have had the opportunity to improve her moral judgment because she was and still is bombarded with the kind of sexist feedback I described. Such feedback is unreliable if it assumes that Eve is incompetent by virtue of being a woman and it is false that most women are morally incompetent. Here, Eve's self-distrust is well grounded because she lacks the relevant competency. Of course, it is important to ensure that evidence for that is not superficial. Sexist norms can cause women to doubt competencies that they do in fact possess. For Eve's attitude to be well grounded, she must actually *be* incompetent, either because of sexism or for some other reason.

Let us now think about what would make Eve's self-distrust justified. She could be incompetent in making important moral decisions while the feedback she receives to her self-distrusting attitudes is reliable in confirming her lack of competence in that domain. In that case, her self-distrust would be well grounded as well as justified. Relevant feedback could be reliable and at the same time motivated by sexist stereotypes if those stereotypes were so damaging that they impeded the development of decision-making skills in most women. Whether feedback imbued with sexism or other forms of oppression is reliable generally speaking depends on the severity of the impact of those norms on oppressed people.

One final case is for Eve's attitude to be justified without it being well grounded. Say that she tends to have reliable attitudes of self-distrust and self-trust, which means that she tends to have the social resources necessary for self-knowledge and to use those resources wisely. However, in this particular case, someone or something in her environment is manipulating her perception of her situation. Someone (e.g., her partner or her physician) might be ensuring that she perceive only evidence of similarities rather than differences between her current situation and situations in the past where she distrusted herself well or trusted herself badly. That scenario may sound familiar, as it is played out in various films. For example, in *The Truman Show*, everyone in the protagonist's social world collaborates to deceive him about the nature of his experience. Similarly, in *Gaslight*, a man nearly convinces his wife that she is crazy by so orchestrating her life that she is cut off from anyone who could confirm her own perceptions. It is possible that deception of that sort is going on in Eve's case, and consequently, that she distrusts herself in a situation in which she would otherwise trust herself. But if she engages in the reliable processes that normally generate her self-distrusting attitudes, her self-distrust would be justified, even though it would not be well grounded.

From a feminist perspective, whether it is reliable to trust or distrust in exceptional cases resembling *The Truman Show* is not as interesting as cases that are influenced by systemic forces of oppression. Reliability is a relative term, indexed to a set of "normal" conditions, that is, conditions in which one can expect a particular event to occur, or, as in the cases I describe, expect someone to be able to develop an attitude that will likely be well grounded.[19] Implicit in my discussion of boundaries of justification for Eve's self-distrust is a certain understanding of what the normal conditions are for her to be justified in distrusting herself. For example, I presumed that the kind of deception she faced in the last example made her situation abnormal. I presumed that the reliability of sexist feedback she received was relative to a set of conditions where women generally either had or had not been so dominated that they embodied the sexist views of their culture. Such feedback together with other manifestations of oppression can make normal conditions for reliable trusting and distrusting relative to various ways in which one is oppressed or privileged.

That aspect of the epistemology of trust is not widely acknowledged. We tend to understand the reliability of trust or distrust only in relation to the privileged case, where normal conditions are normal only for privileged folk. Think again of Jones's example of authoritative and avuncular physicians. By Western standards, they are generally deemed reliable compared with physicians who are hesitant in giving diagnoses, or who are open about the limits of their knowledge of how to care for patients. But how trustworthy the avuncular physician really is depends on who the patient is, and whether the patient is a member of an oppressed group. Most physicians are in a worse position, generally speaking, to understand the health care needs of patients who are oppressed than patients with privilege. They themselves usually live privileged lives that shelter them from the social and environmental constraints on health that many oppressed people face (e.g., barriers posed by poverty, pollution, violence, racism, ableism, etc.). Also physicians' knowledge of how to treat medical conditions that manifest themselves differently among minority groups (especially women) is often vague or incomplete, since members of those groups tend to be excluded or underrepresented as subjects in medical research (Baylis, Downie, and Sherwin 1998). With such gaps in medical knowledge, patients who are oppressed are probably best served by physicians who are honest about the limitations. Since the gaps narrow considerably for people who are multiply privileged (e.g., by class and gender), presumably those patients can trust authoritative and avuncular physicians most of the time.

This illustrates that oppression can make it unsafe, and hence unreliable, for oppressed people to trust others in circumstances in which it is safe for the privileged. (Other examples are seeking police protection in a racist community, and being able to walk alone at night where women are frequently assaulted.) Furthermore, social feedback relevant to one's circumstances can be less reliable for oppressed people compared with those who are comparatively privileged. A man in a similar position as Eve, for example (i.e., making health care decisions that profoundly affect people close to him) may be more likely to have reliable feedback than Eve about whether he can trust himself to do what is right. That is not to say that sexism never distorts a man's self-trusting or self-distrusting attitudes (it can make some men trust themselves too much). However, certainly it can skew those processes to a lesser degree for men or not at all for men compared with women. Think of academic environments in which instructors continually reinforce the sexist view that men's analytic skills are strong whereas those of women are relatively weak (behavior not uncommon among academic instructors; Bartky 1990, 90–93). In classrooms where many men possess those skills but so do many women, and to similar degrees as men, the reliability of feedback will vary along gender lines. As a result, it will be easier for those men than for those women to trust themselves well in academics.

Thus, in evaluating someone's trust or distrust, we have to consider how oppression may have defined the normal conditions for reliable trusting and distrusting for members of that person's social group. Whereas people in privileged positions generally have a good sense of what those conditions are for people "like them," they could cultivate a refined sense of how they differ for people in subordinate positions by learning more about the impact of oppression on those people's lives. That advice is relevant to many health care providers who hope to understand whether the trust or distrust of patients (either in themselves or in their providers) is justified.

Establishing where differences lie in normal conditions for good trusting for members of different social groups also has some emancipatory appeal. For example, it may be unjustified for Eve to trust herself in her situation if the normal conditions for reliable self-trust among women did not allow that (and neither did the feedback she received). However, she would be justified if she were liberated from such an environment. In a new setting in which it was normal for women to trust well in their moral competence, Eve could trust herself with ample justification. Of course, she would have to free herself first of sexist paradigm scenarios for trust and learn to respond positively to nonsexist feedback in her new social environment.

Conclusion and Some Reflection on Eve's Epistemic Autonomy

That last point raises the issue of Eve's epistemic autonomy, which one might think I have ignored thus far. One might worry that sexist feedback seems to have the power to dictate whatever attitudes of self-trust or self-distrust Eve develops. Am I denying her freedom to choose what kind of feedback influences those attitudes? What could epistemic autonomy possibly mean in a theory of trust and distrust where their justification is external to us, where it does not even matter if we acknowledge their justification, and where it involves social, rather than individual, processes?

According to Keith Lehrer (1997), autonomy is required for justified self-trust, which is itself necessary to avoid skepticism about the truth of our beliefs and the "worth" of our desires. "I cannot be worthy of my trust [by which he means that my trust is not justified] if I am not autonomous because, if the evaluations I make are imposed or fortuitous, I have no way of telling whether what I evaluate as worth accepting or preferring is worth accepting or preferring" (Lehrer 1997, 95). Lehrer is an internalist, which is why it is important for him to have a way of telling whether our beliefs or attitudes are justified. That is not important to me as an externalist about trust and distrust, although it is still relevant to me that "the evaluations [we] make [for example, of someone's trustworthiness] are not imposed or fortuitous." Say that an assessment of someone's trustworthiness were imposed on me through brainwashing such that I do not even evaluate the trustworthiness of whoever made that assessment. The resulting attitude could be justified for someone socially positioned as I am if the processes that produced it were reliable in that regard; but since I never engaged in those processes myself I would not be justified in holding that attitude. Distinguishing between an attitude being justified and the bearer of that attitude being justified[20] appears to be necessary in a discussion of epistemic autonomy in an externalist epistemology.

Without moving too deeply into the subject, let me suggest that the autonomy I envision for epistemic subjects who trust or distrust is relational. Feminists devised relational conceptions of autonomy in response to feminist criticism of mainstream conceptions that portray autonomous subjects to be entirely independent or self-sufficient (Meyers 1989; Nedelsky

1989; Code 1991; Friedman 1997; MacKenzie and Stoljar 2000). Their social environments are a potential hindrance to their ability to act on autonomous desires and values. Relational theories of autonomy, by contrast, emphasize not simply how our social relations can interfere with our autonomy, but also how they engender it. To be able to act based on our own beliefs, values, and desires, social resources must be in place that provide us with options to further our values, and with skills to choose autonomously (Meyers 1989; Sherwin 1998). Furthermore, because self-knowledge is social, we require reliable feedback to the process of deciding what we believe, desire, and value. In drawing on that feedback, we do not relinquish our autonomy; nonetheless, we cannot accept the feedback nonreflectively and remain autonomous epistemic agents.

It is the job of the epistemic agent to weed through feedback and discard whatever comes from shady characters or from shady sources generally. Thus, it is only inevitable that sexism would infect Eve's attitudes of self-trust and self-distrust if that were the *only* available feedback (which it was in many examples I described). All epistemic agents have to be careful about what kind of feedback they respond to. Those who learned reliable paradigm scenarios for trust should have little difficulty; however, not everyone learns such scenarios, and not everyone gets feedback laced with good intent rather than a dominating interest. A key point of this chapter is that reliable social feedback of some sort is necessary for having justified attitudes of self-trust and interpersonal trust. We are not free to develop such attitudes otherwise. Oppression can be a formidable barrier there, just as it is to many other kinds of freedoms.

6

The Value of Self-Trust for Autonomy: A Feminist Relational Theory

So far I have established that when we trust ourselves we are optimistic that we will act competently and in accordance with a moral commitment. The commitment can be to promote our own welfare or that of another. It is possible to get things wrong with self-trust because it is an emotional attitude that is cognitive, meaning that it appraises the world in some way and it can do that well or badly. Self-trust is not well-grounded—it represents the world inaccurately—if we are wrong about being competent presently to do what we trust ourselves to do and about being committed to doing it with moral integrity. Getting things wrong while trusting ourselves can cause harm or disappointment to ourselves and others when we fail to meet our moral commitments. Getting things wrong in distrusting ourselves can cause harm to us, as it can reinforce low levels of self-respect and prevent us from seizing new opportunities. People who are psychologically oppressed or abused are especially vulnerable to such harm or disappointment.

In this chapter I focus on why it is important to gets things right with self-trust and self-distrust. The answer lies in the connection between trusting oneself well and being an autonomous agent. Autonomy is a property of agents who act in a particular way (or a property of actions insofar as they are committed by agents who act autonomously). People who have autonomy reflect on what they truly believe and value, and they act accordingly. They are also competent and committed to engage in such reflection and to act on the results. Furthermore, they have a positive attitude toward their own competency and commitment. In other words, they trust themselves to make an autonomous decision (Govier

1993b). Such an attitude is "not to be taken for granted," for "[it] can be put in question by challenges—either from other people or from the course of events" (Govier 1993b, 112). I expand on and refine Govier's theory that self-trust is important for autonomy, and add to it a feminist analysis of the challenges that many people face to their potential to be self-trusting. Moreover, since I interpret self-trust as a moral attitude toward the self (unlike Govier), I maintain that the autonomy it promotes has a moral dimension. All autonomous action has such a dimension, in my view, and therefore self-trust is crucial for all autonomous behavior.

I also consider whether just any agent who trusts herself is autonomous. Govier stated that those who trust themselves too much are not autonomous (1993b, 115). I specify what "too much" means by concluding that to have autonomy we must be able to develop justified attitudes of self-trust, and we must exercise that ability.[1] Knowing how to distrust our selves well is no trivial matter for autonomy either; however, too much self-distrust of any kind is detrimental to our autonomy. Attitudes of self-trust and self-distrust are justified if the psychological and social processes generating them are reliable. For autonomy, we need reliable self-trusting and self-distrusting attitudes most of the time; we do not have to get things right all of the time.

Justified self-trust is important for autonomy, but some autonomy is also important for justified self-trust; at the end of chapter 5, I noted that some epistemic autonomy is necessary for being justified in trusting oneself. Hence, the relation between self-trust and autonomy is reciprocal, not unidirectional. I join Keith Lehrer (1997) in acknowledging the value of autonomy for self-trust, although I interpret what autonomy means and what the conditions are that promote it differently.

Understanding the reciprocal relation between autonomy and self-trust is important because of the value of autonomy apart from that relation. Where is the value in being autonomous? The answer lies partly in the disvalue of oppression, exploitation, and abuse. People who do not have adequate autonomy skills are particularly vulnerable to the subtle workings of oppression and other forms of injustice. Thus, endorsing an ethical principle of respect for the autonomy of others has emancipatory appeal, particularly in contexts where a heightened threat of abuse or coercion exists. Autonomy is not about mere absence of threats to the self, however. In concert with others (Meyers' 1989; Dworkin 1989; Young 1989), I hold that people who are autonomous set goals for themselves that give their lives purpose. Autonomy is essential, in other words, for human flourishing (Stoljar 1996).

Despite its emancipatory appeal, the ideal of autonomy is contentious in feminist circles. Feminists have claimed that the ideal favors the traditionally masculine trait of self-sufficiency and that it is built on a conception of the self as unified and presocial.[2] Such a conception is absurd from the perspective of many women who experience themselves in ways that highlight the degree to which their selves are shaped by numerous and often competing social forces.

Feminist criticism is directed in part toward a caricature of autonomy found in libertarian theory as well as in cultural icons, such as the "self-made man" or the Marlboro man (Friedman 1997; Mackenzie and Stoljar 2000). However, the criticism also targets liberal conceptions of autonomy that treat "the individual as ontologically prior to the social" (Young 1990, 45). Many feminists share with communitarians a view of the self as unremittingly social (Friedman 1997); that is, "a product of social processes, not their origin" (Young 1990, 45). Unlike most communitarians, however, feminists include among those social processes the political processes of oppression. The feminist social self is a sociopolitical self.

Some feminists have revived the ideal of autonomy and made it consistent with the sociopolitical dimensions of selfhood. Together with some nonfeminists (Taylor 1985) they defend relational conceptions of autonomy that emphasize not only how the social aspects of persons interfere potentially with their ability to be autonomous, but also how they engender that ability (Mackenzie and Stoljar 2000). A uniquely feminist project is to identify what the political aspects of persons imply about the kinds of social relations that either hinder or promote our autonomy. In previous chapters I undertook a similar project about self-trust and developed a feminist relational theory of justified attitudes of self-trust and self-distrust. My theory of the importance of those attitudes for autonomy is clearly situated within the frame of feminist relational autonomy theory.

Some feminists have expanded that frame to include the field of bioethics (Sherwin 1998; McLeod and Sherwin 2000; Donchin 1995 2000; Dodds 2000). I join them here by grounding my analysis of the value of self-trust for autonomy in some patients' experiences with infertility treatment. Oppressive norms about women's reproductivity make the threat of self-distrust particularly severe for female patients compared with male patients in fertility clinics.

Standard versus Relational Theories of Autonomy: How the Former Pathologize the Nonautonomous Subject

Let me begin by outlining the contribution of feminist relational approaches to contemporary autonomy theory, and by offering some feminist criticism of standard theories in moral philosophy and bioethics. In general, those theories are not susceptible to the feminist charge of being individualistic, in the sense of prescribing an ideal of self-sufficiency. They tend to acknowledge that autonomy is consistent with maintaining personal relationships (Beauchamp and Childress 1994; Dworkin 1989). Nonetheless, standard theories have an implicit presumption that one is somehow "pathological or infantile" if one is neither autonomous nor subject to explicit coercion or manipulation.[3] Standard conceptions *are* individualistic in the sense that they ignore (or deny) the full extent to which power relations in our society can undermine our autonomy. I make that point as I outline what those theories say about the basic conditions for autonomy as well as potential obstacles to those conditions. I then show the contrast offered by feminist relational theories, which describe oppression as a substantial threat to autonomy.

Theorists of autonomy in mainstream bioethics and moral philosophy do not all agree on the conditions necessary for autonomy. Without presuming agreement among them, I construct a list of conditions that draws together their many contributions to contemporary autonomy theory. The list includes, broadly speaking, that we are able to make choices based on our own desires, beliefs, and values (level of choice), that we can act on those choices (level of action), and that the forces influencing our mental attitudes are not alien to the self (level of authenticity).

Choice
To be able to choose based on our own beliefs, desires, and values, bioethicists say that we require decisional capacity, or competence, as well as

adequate understanding of our options (Beauchamp and Childress 1994; Faden and Beauchamp 1986). Decisional capacity allows us to understand the nature of our options and to evaluate them in light of our beliefs and values. Clearly, to be in a position to exercise that capacity, we must be adequately informed. In settings where it is unlikely that we would have the relevant information ready at hand (such as health care settings), it is important that someone disclose information about our options to us. Bioethicists acknowledge that inadequate disclosure and poor communication by health care providers is a potential obstacle to understanding. Yet they also highlight the "limited knowledge bases" of some patients (Beauchamp and Childress 1994, 158). For many bioethicists, as well as mainstream moral philosophers, ignorance is a primary obstacle to autonomy.[4]

Bioethicists tend not to specify which attitudes should inform our choices. However, not just any attitudes will do since some of them may conflict and some we may hold only fleetingly. An adequate theory of autonomy must explain how we sort through incompatible desires, beliefs, and values when choosing autonomously. We do that, according to some moral philosophers, by engaging in reflection at a "second-order level" and by acting on whichever attitudes we identify with at that level (Dworkin 1989; Frankfurt 1989). If we act, instead, on our first-order beliefs, desires, and values without accepting them as our own, we relinquish our autonomy. We become "wantons," people who are not concerned about "whether the desires that move [them] to act are desires by which [they want] to be moved to act" (Frankfurt 1989, 68). Wantonness, weakness of will, as well as brainwashing and posthypnotic suggestion are the main obstacles to "identification" in standard theories of autonomy in moral philosophy.

Meyers (1989) and mainstream moral theorist Robert Young (1989) emphasize the importance for autonomy of acting in accordance with a "life plan." Autonomy is about self-direction, but we cannot be self-directed unless some sort of plan guides our action. In fact, what partly explains why we identify with certain attitudes is that they further the plan we have for our lives. Now one might balk at the idea of having a life plan, especially if one's life is perpetually disorganized. However, the kinds of life plans that are conducive to autonomy can be ill defined at least with respect to some areas of our lives, and they can also (and probably should) be continually under revision (Meyers 1989, 49; 2000, 172). According to Young, on the other hand, to have the type of plan necessary for autonomy, we must have brought "the entire course of [our lives] into a unified order" (1989, 78).⁵ Young labels a person "anomic" who falls to organize his life and the maxims guiding his behavior in a unified way.

Action

Being in a position to make choices that reflect our life plans, as well as the beliefs and values with which we identify, is not sufficient for autonomy. A second broad condition is that we must be free to act on the choices *we* make, as opposed to choices made for us by others. Thus, moral philosophers acknowledge that coercion is an obstacle to autonomy (e.g., Dworkin 1989; Christman 1991), and bioethicists say that "voluntariness" is an essential criterion (Beauchamp and Childress 1994; Faden and Beauchamp 1986). The latter rightly insist that patients' decisions be voluntary, meaning free of coercion and manipulation. Yet they tend to define coercion so narrowly that it includes only explicit forms that are directed "toward (or away from) one of [the patient's] options" (Sherwin 1998, 26). Coercive forces can be subtler than that and they can have a broader target, such as a patient's appreciation for her own competence in making decisions. That point is missing from the work of most mainstream bioethicists and moral philosophers. One would have to conclude, in their theories, that patients who are influenced by social norms and stereotypes that challenge their decisional capacity are not coerced, they are simply weak willed.

   Let me explain briefly why undermining a person's appreciation for her decisional capacity often amounts to coercion. I coerce you "when I so manipulate your circumstances that you have fewer options than before, and the best of them, X, which is what I want you to do, is one you would not have chosen in the prethreat situation" (Campbell 1998, 185). If I so manipulate you that you do not feel capable of making many decisions on your own, the best option for you will be to defer to my authority. Doing otherwise *confidently* is no longer an option. Therefore, in an important sense, your options have decreased. I have coerced you if deferring to me or if what I choose on your behalf is not what you would have chosen in the "prethreat situation." Note that the "I" does not have to be a conscious, deliberate agent. "You" can be coerced by the entire institutional structure of a society and by the social norms embedded within it.

The requirement that we have some appreciation for our capacity to be autonomous is a substantive condition for autonomy, unlike conditions such as engaging in self-reflection at a second-order level, which are purely procedural. Most standard theories of autonomy are purely procedural. They oblige us to subject our first-order mental attitudes to some procedure or method of evaluation and act on whatever attitudes satisfy the procedure. But they do not require us to believe or value anything specific in order to be autonomous (Benson 1994, 653). Bioethical theories are somewhat of an exception, as they emphasize the condition of understanding, which limits what patients can believe about the nature of their health care options if they are to choose autonomously. That condition is substantive, not procedural, because it restricts the content (specifically, the factual, not the normative content) of an autonomous agent's mental attitudes. Feminist theorists Robin Dillon (1992, 1997) and Paul Benson (1994) have endorsed the substantive condition that autonomous agents have some self-respect and self-worth, respectively. Below, I support their theories and introduce my own substantive condition of justified self-trust.

Authenticity

A third broad condition for autonomy can be found in the work of some moral philosophers, such as Young (1989) and Christman (1989, 1991). They propose that the manner in which our goals and second-order attitudes are formed is also relevant. To be autonomous, we have to define our goals and values for ourselves, rather than simply accept what others want for us. This involves discovering what we ourselves believe and value, and defining ourselves accordingly.[6] Thus, Meyers (1989) noted that self-definition and self-discovery (i.e., self-understanding) are as important for autonomy as self-direction. Although Meyers did not acknowledge it as such, self-understanding is a substantive condition for autonomy, for surely we can be wrong about what our selves are like. Potential sources of error within standard theories of autonomy are rooted almost entirely in the self; examples are neuroses and self-deception.

Standard theories of autonomy in bioethics and moral philosophy have contributed greatly to our understanding of autonomy; but, at the same time, they have misled us about what the primary obstacles are. I agree that the broad conditions above are important, but I disagree that more often than not, some pathology or weakness in the agent explains their absence. It appears that for mainstream moral philosophers, paradigms of the heteronomous subject are the neurotic, the anomic, and the wanton; they depict that subject as pathologically weak-willed, self-deceived, or simply pathological. Furthermore, they reinforce that impression by narrowly defining external sources of heteronomy, restricting them beyond explicit coercion to such unusual cases as brainwashing and posthypnotic suggestion. Bioethicists similarly give a narrow description of those sources, although they often do blame physicians for limiting the autonomy of patients. The external barriers to autonomy that they and most moral philosophers ignore are oppressive and abusive social relations.

An adequate theory must account for the ways in which oppression and abuse can interfere with the various conditions necessary for autonomy. Following Susan Sherwin (1998) and Catriona Mackenzie (2000, 114), I will explain how oppression threatens each of those conditions.

Oppression and Choice

Being socialized in an oppressive way can limit one's ability to choose well by hindering development of skills necessary to make choices in light of one's own beliefs, values, and goals. Autonomy demands a "repertory of skills," including those of "discern[ing] the import of felt self-referential responses [i.e., one's attraction or repulsion to different options]," and of resisting unwanted pressure from others (Meyers 1989, 81, 84; 2000, 166). Acquisition of such skills can be blocked or delayed through the influence of oppressive stereotypes, such as of women's diminished capacity for autonomy. Part of the lore of most patriarchal cultures is that women are naturally dependent on the approval of others and are disinclined to make choices that further their own interests (Meyers 1989, 142; Bartky 1990, 24, 25). The truth is that many women are *taught* to "over-identify with others' interests and to neglect their own"

(Meyers 1989, 143). In extreme cases, they do not even learn how to discern what their own interests are by evaluating their self-referential responses. Sexist socialization can severely restrict the opportunities for women to develop autonomy skills.

Oppression is also a factor at the level at which choices are made because it can ensure that members of oppressed groups are not situated to choose as well as those who are comparatively privileged, having less of the information they require to make such choices. In the context of health care delivery, information available to patients is limited to whatever research has been conducted and to whatever individual health care providers assume is relevant to their patients (Sherwin 1998, 27). Rarely does medical research cover gender differences in the manifestation, prevalence, and treatment of different illnesses, and (to make matters worse for women) it is sometimes conducted exclusively on male subjects (Baylis, Downie, and Sherwin 1998, 238). Thus, the information gathered does not necessarily put women in an equal position to men for choosing autonomously in health care contexts.

Patients also rely on individual health care providers to inform them of benefits and harms associated with different procedures; and yet often what constitutes a harm or a benefit is relative to one's social position. The social standpoint especially of patients who experience several forms of oppression (such as racism, poverty, and ableism) tends to differ dramatically from that of health care providers (Sherwin 1998, 27). Consequently, there are either barriers to effective communication or patients simply fail to receive the information they require to further their own interests.

Oppression and Action
Oppression can interfere at the level of one's ability to act on one's choices. If relevant choices oppose one's oppression, one might not have the courage to act on them or might have lingering desires, with which one does not fully identify, that conflict with those choices. Consider a woman who was taught that a woman's greatest asset is her looks. After years of going to great lengths to conform to society's beauty standards, she decides to throw out her hot rollers and her drawer full of make-up, and cancel next week's appointment for a facial and waxing. She is sick

of spending so much time (and money) trying to make herself look "beautiful." But soon she starts to regret her decision, not because she reevaluates whether her looks define her worth, but because of the rewards she has given up, which for her include respect and attention at work by those who control the advancement of her career. She is in a classic double-bind, where the likely consequences of choosing either option (conforming or not conforming) are harmful (Morgan 1991). Oppressed people tend to find themselves in such situations disproportionately compared with the privileged (Frye 1983), and hence it is more common for them to confront obstacles to their ability to act on their choices.

Double-binds are significant barriers to choosing autonomously, but they are not necessarily insurmountable. People with advanced autonomy skills can often reconcile competing desires (Meyers 2000, 170). Yet notice the paradox when they are from oppressed groups. Oppression demands superior autonomy skills by proliferating double-binds, and at the same time limits opportunities for developing such skills.

Oppression can interfere at the level of acting autonomously also by ensuring that whatever option would further one's desires or goals does not exist. The autonomy of minority groups in health care contexts can be limited because the option they prefer (or would prefer) is "prematurely excluded" (Sherwin 1998, 26). For example, that is normally the case for lesbians who might choose a high-tech means of assisted reproduction to have a genetically related child if they had that option.[7] Members of minority groups commonly find themselves in such a position because they are underrepresented on institutional bodies that make policy decisions about which options should be available (Sherwin 1998, 27).

Oppression and Authenticity

Oppression can shape the desires and goals of oppressed people in ways that limit their autonomy (Friedman 1986; Babbitt 1996; MacKenzie 2000). It can so influence their self-concepts or identities that they adopt goals and values that further their own oppression. For example, a woman who is infertile may have learned to identify so strongly with pregnancy and motherhood that she is willing to do whatever it takes to conceive, even subjecting herself continually to treatments that she finds emotionally and physically harmful. Often, oppression encourages nonautonomous goals and values by diminishing self-respect and self-worth (Dillon 1992, 1997; Benson 1994). A person who is psychologically oppressed may feel that she is not worthy of respectful treatment. The life goals, desires, and values with which she identifies reflect that self-conception. But to say that she suffers from some pathology is disrespectful, as it implies that the fault lies within her. In her case, social pathology, rather than an individual pathology, interferes with the formation of her goals, desires, and values.

Oppression is therefore a potential barrier to each of the conditions necessary for autonomy. Nonetheless, the actual barrier it poses to each oppressed person varies significantly. Not everyone who is oppressed internalizes oppressive norms or is denied the opportunity to develop autonomy skills (Sherwin 1998, 37, 38). Some oppressed people (e.g., some black or First Nations people) live in proud, culturally vibrant communities that tend to foster autonomy skills in their members. And although women rarely have such communities of their own (Bartky 1990, 25), they often come close to creating them with women's collectives. Furthermore, many women are situated in overlapping spheres of oppression and privilege, and consequently experience some of the ways in which privilege can enhance autonomy. For example, a woman with middle-class privilege could strengthen her capacities for understanding and critical reflection by receiving an excellent education. Privilege, however, is not an unqualified good in the domain of autonomy. The beliefs and values of a middle-class woman may be unwittingly influenced by classist norms, which she might regard as alien to her.

Autonomy is therefore relational in the sense that it requires a nonoppressive social environment that builds or fosters autonomy skills. Below, I maintain that autonomy is even more relational than that because of the value of justified self-trust and the profoundly relational way in which such attitudes develop.

Oppression-Related and Paralytic Self-Distrust: The Context of Infertility Treatment

The various ways in which oppression can negatively affect women's autonomy are present in the context of modern infertility treatment.

Proponents of these technologies claim that they enhance the autonomy of some women (and some men) by offering them choices that hitherto were unavailable (Robertson 1994); however, many feminists have shown the weaknesses in those arguments. For example, social norms, such as those of pronatalism, make it extremely difficult for women to refuse assisted reproductive technologies (ARTs) upon discovering that they are infertile (Shanner 1996; Morgan 1989). Such norms and other mechanisms of oppression can prevent women and men who struggle with infertility from trusting themselves to make autonomous decisions in that domain. Drawing on experiences of some patients undergoing infertility treatment, I maintain that self-distrust is an obstacle to autonomy that is often tied to oppression.

Self-distrust can occur at all three levels at which oppression can interfere with autonomy: people can distrust that they will choose well or that they will act on the choices they make, and they can distrust their judgment about which attitudes should inform their choices.

Self-Distrust and Choice

To trust that they will choose well, people must be able to rely on their skills in making choices, to rely on information they use to make choices, and to trust sources of that information. People will find it difficult to rely on their autonomy skills if oppressive social conditions have stunted the development of those skills. Yet even if they have acquired the necessary skills, they may feel pessimistic about their ability to choose autonomously because of what society has taught them to expect of their abilities. Even though they may have been successful in the past in making good decisions, they might interpret those successes as flukes, and suspect that at any moment someone will expose them as fakes.

Of course, a person need not feel like a fake or distrust herself in every domain as a result of oppression. Distrust in one's ability to choose well can be domain specific if it is motivated by oppressive stereotypes that target specific competencies. For example, poor people with little formal education are stereotyped as incompetent in making decisions that involve abstract reasoning, but not in deciding how to treat others respectfully, how to perform manual tasks, and so on. Alternatively, stereotypes that engender domain-specific self-distrust can target the expertise of a particular social group, rather than the (in)competency of another. Physicians are stereotyped (positively from their perspective) as wise and thoughtful decision makers on all kinds of health care matters, including those that are not primarily medical. A patient who is given the option of using ARTs might distrust her ability to choose well while in the company of a physician who she feels is more qualified to make the decision.

Sometimes self-distrust is appropriate, but where it is not and it persists, it forms a barrier to autonomy. Distrusting one's ability to choose well in domains where one has frequently made bad decisions in the past is appropriate. Still, it can paralyze one from making choices at all or it can cause one to defer continually to the judgment of others. "With the self in default, something else would take over. Perhaps one would be governed by others—a parent, husband, or charismatic leader" (Govier 1993, 108). The others might govern benevolently or simply manipulate one to fulfil *their* desires, which would be easy, since one prefers not to choose on one's own anyway.

To trust that one will choose well, one also has to be able to rely on information that is relevant to the choice and to trust the purveyor of that information. In infertility treatment, the relevant information can be inordinately complex or hopelessly vague. Complexity due to the sheer number of options available can make decisions inherently difficult. For example, woman may be asked to decide whether they want to continue taking so-called fertility drugs (i.e., ovulation-induction agents), to try ovarian hyperstimulation,[8] or to go with something more high-tech, such as in vitro fertilization (IVF). They also may have other options, such as IVF coupled with intra cytoplasmic sperm injection (ICSI), where sperm are injected into the ova.[9] With each option, the likelihood of conception increases, but so does the financial cost and potential health risks. Given the difficulty of weighing such risks, costs, and success rates of different procedures, women may distrust their judgment about which decision is best for them. Consequently, they may pick up on any suggestion by their physician about what they should do, and go with that. Their inclination to defer to the physician because they distrust their own judgment interferes with them being able to make an autonomous choice, a choice based their own values and goals, rather than those of the physician.

Vagueness is a problem with some of the information patients receive. Since many forms of ART are still experimental, the risks involved are largely unknown. Many women undergoing IVF soon discover that neither good evidence nor straight answers are forthcoming about their risks of cancer and other long-term side effects (Shanner 1996, 130). Concerns about cancer arise in connection with drugs that suppress or stimulate ovulation, and they extend to the health of the potential future child.[10]

Furthermore, physicians sometimes refuse to give straight answers about the success rates of their fertility clinics. Much controversy has surrounded that issue in Canada, where most clinics do not publicize live birth rates. Instead, they quote universal data about the success of a procedure generally or in Canada specifically. Such data are misleading because success rates in Canada are often much lower than in the United States, and they can vary substantially among Canadian clinics.[11]

Patients are also not always adequately informed about what an emotional roller-coaster infertility treatment can be, which is especially true for women in IVF programs. Those patients undergo frequent hormone injections and frequent and invasive physical examinations, and they can be cancelled[12] from the program at any moment for "failing" to ovulate or because embryos do not implant in their uterus.[13] As one woman who was quoted in the Canadian media said, "It was like going to a used-car dealership. You had no idea what you were getting into" (*Globe and Mail,* May 22, 1999, A9). Some but not all[14] clinics have counselors who will describe the emotional aspects of treatment and provide support to patients. However, as employees of the clinics themselves, they have dual loyalties to patients and to physicians, and their relationships with patients are compromised as a result. Many patients, understandably, would feel uncomfortable expressing their concerns about the emotional strain of treatment to counselors who have some allegiance to the program's physicians (i.e., to those who are committed to the treatments being helpful, not harmful).

Some patients find it difficult to rely on the information they receive about ART because they distrust the service providers. Moreover, their distrust may be connected with their sociopolitical position relative to the position of most physicians. "Considering the history of sickle-cell screening, the Tuskegee syphilis experiment, and other medical abuses, many Blacks harbour a well-founded distrust of technological interference with their bodies and genetic material at the hands of white physicians" (Roberts 1997, 260). That may be one reason why black people are half as likely as white people to use high-tech means of treating infertility (other reasons have to do with culture and economics; Roberts 1997, 251). Most babies conceived by ARTs are white.

If, for whatever reason, patients cannot rely on information they receive about ARTs, but they trust a decision to use those technologies nonetheless, their decision may not be fully autonomous. As I mentioned, not all forms of self-distrust inhibit autonomy, and conversely, not all forms of self-trust promote autonomy. Choices that are autonomous are meant to further our goals and interests, but choices with many unexpected consequences can have the opposite effect of subverting our interests. Granted, at times we might value choosing for its own sake, in which case the consequences are irrelevant to whether the choice is autonomous. But usually we make choices for the sake of achieving a certain outcome, which is especially true in the case of infertility treatment, where the preferred outcome is a genetically related child.

Consequences relevant to whether a choice in favor of infertility treatment is autonomous usually extend beyond the success of the procedures, however. There is a limit to what most patients are willing to go through to have a genetically related child; most do not have the attitude of doing whatever it takes (despite how the media tend to portray them). For example, it is not clear that Joanne was willing to go as far as IVF took her to have a child. She trusted her decision knowing that the process would be difficult emotionally, but since she had been successful in the past in dealing with many hardships, she assumed that she could cope. Still, she never expected that IVF would be as difficult as it was: "It was so bad, so stressful. And I consider myself pretty good at coping with things usually. But at one point . . . honest to God I almost packed up and left. I thought, 'I cannot stand this another second.' It was like a time capsule of all of your expectations and all of your stress just jam packed into five days or six days or whatever it was. And you never got any relief from it" (Williams 1989, 136).[15] It may be that Joanne simply overestimated her ability to cope or she was never properly informed about how emotionally draining an IVF cycle can be. Either way, her choice was not fully autonomous, since she suffered extreme and unexpected consequences that undermined the value she placed in her own well-being.

Self-Distrust and Action

When Joanne "almost packed up and left," she may have decided that was the right thing to do; however, she did not act on that decision because she lacked self-trust. Trusting ourselves to act on our choices is crucial for autonomy; but with ARTs, factors relating to women's oppression can inhibit that trust. We live in a culture of "obligatory fertility" for women (Morgan 1989, 70),[16] where women who are infertile are supposedly diseased and those who choose to be childless are selfish or crazy. Feminists who insist that ARTs limit women's choices point to the ease with which they allow others to judge women who are infertile but who choose not to have or not to continue with infertility treatments (Royal Commission 1993, 37). When women stop the treatment or choose not to start it, they are subject to the stigma of "voluntary childlessness" (Shanner 1996, 131). Worry over that stigma might explain in part why Lois behaved as she did on discovering that she had been cancelled from an IVF program because she had ovulated before her ova could be retrieved: "I remember getting in the car and crying all the way home. I'm never going back there. They've had enough! I'm not a guinea pig any more! (she laughs nervously) And I was just . . . I'd had it. I thought—this is it. I'm not doing this again. But about two days afterwards it was, okay, let's go back in (she laughs)" (Williams 1989, 130). If one views Lois's choice to go back without reflecting on the social context, one might assume that she is masochistic or perhaps even schizophrenic. A more charitable interpretation is that Lois cannot trust herself to act on a decision to end treatment because not only might that make her childless, it would imply that she chose to be that way.

While undergoing infertility treatment, some patients might distrust themselves to voice and therefore to act on a decision about how treatment should proceed. They might fear that if they go against physicians' recommendations or object to the way physicians are performing procedures they will be labeled "noncompliant" and uncooperative, and as a result will lose the support of care providers. Recall Lee from the Introduction. She strongly objected to what was happening during the hysteroscopy; however, getting off the operating table and leaving the room would have given her providers additional reason for viewing her as a "problem patient."

Some people might distrust themselves to act on a choice to enter a fertility program at all if they are aware of some of the complexities it involves, such as how it might reinforce a sexist perception of women's social role and the concept of infertility as a disease. Some women might be eminently aware of the restricted access of treatment to couples who can afford it, and usually to women who are heterosexual and married. They might know that many disadvantaged women in North America and elsewhere do not even have access to basic reproductive health care services (Royal Commission 1992, 38, 39), and some are subject to welfare reform measures that are designed to prevent their reproduction (Roberts 1997, 269). In other words, prospective patients may understand that a choice in favor of infertility treatment is not purely personal (Sherwin 1992); it lends support to a certain stereotype of women as well as to an unfair distribution of health care resources.[17] At the same time, to assume that people drawn to that choice are extraordinarily selfish is both unkind and unfair. All of their lives, they may have pictured having a child, and now they face continual reminders in the media and elsewhere about how empty their lives must be. In the end, some of them might trust that a decision to use ARTs is right for them because of the pain of childlessness, yet still have lingering desires to avoid perpetuating injustice.

Self-Distrust and Authenticity

The double-binds of infertility in a pronatalist, high-tech culture can promote self-distrust at the level of one's judgment about the beliefs, values, and desires that influence one's choices. A woman who is infertile might wonder how autonomous her desire for a child is because of the obvious connection between that desire and the gender socialization of women. She might question the choice to enter a fertility program because of how it could further her oppression, especially given the severe emotional and physical stress it can entail. Lois's sudden reversal in her position on further infertility treatment could be the result of distrust in her own judgment on which desires, beliefs, and values should inform that position.

Distrust at the level of one's judgment can also arise because of the feeling of being objectified in treatment. Having your body exposed, palpitated, and prodded, often by people unknown to you, can easily cause such feelings. Lee eventually linked her objectification with feelings of confusion and uncertainty about what she needed and deserved. The more objectified she felt, the more confused she became. Such a response is explicable on an understanding of objectification as a form of "psychic alienation," or "estrangement . . . of a person from some of the essential attributes of personhood" (Bartky 1990, 30). Objectification causes such estrangement by reducing a person to the status of parts of her that are inessential to her personhood, such as her sexual or reproductive parts (Bartky 1990, 26). It makes sense that feeling separated from what makes one a person would promote confusion about whether one truly deserves to have one's opinions heard and to be treated respectfully.

Patients might distrust their judgment about whether feelings of objectification are even justified because of forces in our culture that normalize the kinds of medical interventions they find objectifying. Whereas they might sense that the interventions treat women as mere "reproductive vessels," they might also assume that it is "normal" for women to seek medical treatment for infertility (even though it is generally normal only for white, middle-class, heterosexual women). Consider this man's response when his partner had her ova removed during an IVF cycle: " . . . all of a sudden I'm in the Twilight Zone. It's not a hospital, it's a . . . garage! And my wife is the car and these are the grease monkeys, down to the bad radio blaring and the power tools. I feel a surge of anger at this; how could they treat my wife's body as if it were a machine? Then I waver—no; it's just that they've done this so many times it is mechanical for them. It shows confidence, not disrespect. After all, I'm in their shop" (Mentor 1998, 68). Mentor is clearly influenced as well by sexist norms that physicians who are overconfident (that is, who display masculine characteristics of strength and certainty regarding their behavior) are more reliable than physicians who are more cautious (see chapter 5; Jones 1996, 21). Such norms, together with societal expectations about what is normal for the treatment of women in reproductive medicine, can influence patients' values and beliefs to the point at which they seem alien to the self.

Thus in the context of infertility treatment barriers such as oppression-related double binds and inadequate information can cause patients to distrust that they will choose and act autonomously. Although some of those factors (e.g., inadequate information) can arise in other medical contexts as well, the context of reproductive medicine is the one that poses barriers to women's self-trust that are connected with their oppressed reproductive roles. Women contemplating infertility treatment have to weigh their options in light of not only incomplete information but also complex pronatalist expectations that reinforce sexist oppression. Pronatalist forces can threaten self-trust to such a point that the patient is paralyzed or forced to defer to the judgment of others. Self-distrust of such an extreme sort clearly compromises autonomy.

However, not all of the ways in which patients might distrust themselves in infertility treatment contexts interfere with their autonomy. Women might distrust that choosing ARTs is consistent with their moral values, and worry legitimate about acting on a choice that might subvert those values. Self-distrust bars them, at least temporarily, from acting in a way that could undermine their autonomy.

Thus, self-distrust is a potential threat to autonomy, but not necessarily an actual threat. That point does not establish, however, that self-trust is necessary for autonomy, as someone could lack self-distrust and yet not be self-trusting. Drawing on Karen Jones, I explained in chapter 2 that trust and distrust are contraries, but not contradictories, which means that one could be merely indifferent toward one's own trustworthiness. Autonomous agents must be more than just indifferent in that regard. To have the will to be autonomous, they must be optimistic about their competence and commitment to make decisions that reflect their values and interests. Thus, to be autonomous is to have self-trust of some sort.

But why should self-trust be the self-regarding attitude that describes our will to be autonomous? Furthermore, if it is the relevant attitude, and if I am right that it is a moral attitude toward the self, does that not imply that all autonomous decisions have a moral dimension? Can we not choose and act autonomously in spheres that are nonmoral?

The Moral Dimension of Autonomy

I claim, in opposition to Meyers (1989) specifically that all autonomous decisions have a moral aspect; and therefore, self-trust can be the self-regarding attitude that motivates us to be autonomous. In choosing and acting autonomously, we strive to meet moral responsibilities to the self, to others, or to both. We are optimistic about fulfilling those responsibilities when we trust ourselves at each of the three levels of decision making I discussed.

Meyers acknowledged the importance of having the will to act autonomously. She noted that two "volitional modes" are necessary for autonomy: resistance to unwarranted pressure from others and resolve, which "is a person's determination to act on his or her own judgments" (1989, 83). The resolve criterion overlaps with my criterion of trusting oneself to act on one's choices, although resolve and self-trust are not identical. One can resolve to do something that has no moral significance (e.g., becoming good at Nintendo), whereas one does not trust oneself to do something unless it is, in some sense, moral.

But do autonomous acts always have moral significance? The standard answer in moral philosophy is "no," and Meyers concurred. The category of "personal autonomy," she claimed, encompasses a wider range of behavior than "moral autonomy" (1989, 13–19), where the latter refers to self-regulating behavior that is consistent with the agent's own "moral sense" (1987).[18] Some autonomous decisions are purely personal; that is true ordinarily of the choice of someone as one's spouse, for example (Meyers 1989, 15). However, no one type of decision is always purely personal. Whether one chooses a particular person as one's spouse becomes a moral matter if "one has actively [and voluntarily] encouraged a suitor to think that his or her love is returned and that a proposal of marriage would be accepted" (Meyers 1989, 15). It becomes a moral matter when refusing would violate one's duties to the person who proposed. The kinds of decisions that one can make without violating one's moral autonomy are limited by the class of actions that one deems to be morally permissible. In other words, moral autonomy determines "the outer bounds" of personal autonomy (Meyers 1989, 14).

It is conceivable that those outer bounds are purely procedural. In other words, there may be procedural restrictions only (as opposed to procedural and substantive restrictions) on our moral autonomy, such as the Kantian restriction that rules governing our behavior be universalizable; that is, applicable to any agent in relevantly similar circumstances (Meyers 1989, 13). In that case, as long as we dutifully follow the procedure of universalizing the maxims for our action, those maxims are in fact moral and we are morally autonomous in living up to them.

Although conceivable, a purely procedural theory of moral autonomy is unconvincing. Horrendous types of behavior can satisfy most procedural restrictions; as Meyers wrote, someone could "sincerely universalize the most despicable practices" (Meyers 1987, 150; 1994, chapter 2). In her view, therefore, substantive limits must exist on the kinds of values that morally autonomous agents can have. I endorsed such a limit in accepting that they must appreciate their own worth, which means that they must be somewhat responsible to themselves.

Meyers formally accepted the substantive restriction that moral responsibilities to the self should guide the behavior of autonomous agents (1989, 17; 1987, 152); however, many of her examples of choices that are "purely personal" concerned whether someone was fulfilling such responsibilities. For example, once we acknowledge that duties to the self exist, it is hard to imagine why a choice of someone as one's spouse would not ordinarily have a moral dimension. There may be instances in which that choice is purely personal, such as when one has to choose between two people and either choice would fulfil one's responsibilities to them and to oneself; but surely, they are atypical. Normally, it is not a moot issue whether in choosing someone as one's spouse, one is being "true to [oneself]—[to one's] own needs and desires" (Meyers 1987, 152), which is how Meyers interpreted duties to the self. On that interpretation, it is difficult to see why many of her examples fall outside of the purview of morality. Consider the struggle of "Ibsen's Nora . . . to break out of her husband's stifling emotional grip and also out of her society's hold on her apprehension of her proper role" (Meyers 1989, 19). Surely, someone in Nora's position, if she is able, should be more attentive to her needs and desires, rather than focused predominantly on others' needs. To stand up for what we ourselves need is part and parcel of appreciating our own worth.

Thus, Meyers formally set up a distinction between personal and moral autonomy, but it became blurred in her examples of personally autonomous and personally nonautonomous decisions. She may want to preserve that distinction nonetheless for the following reason. We tend to deal with situations in which people neglect their responsibilities to themselves very differently than those in which they fail to meet their responsibilities to others. We do not often feel (nor should we) that we have the moral standing to judge people's own decisions about what is best for them, whereas we moralize all of the time about people's decisions that directly concern the welfare of others. Judging people openly for how well they live up to their responsibilities to themselves is not only inappropriate in many circumstances, it can also be harmful if it amounts to victim blaming as it might in a case like Nora's (Meyers, personal communication). Given that we do approach people's decisions for themselves differently from their decisions for others, maintaining the distinction, personal versus moral autonomy, seems to be in order.

I have two objections to that view. One is that saying "personal versus moral" obscures the fact that moral responsibilities to the self exist and play an important role in autonomous decision making. Second, moralizing about how well people treat themselves is sometimes justified: specifically, where one does have the moral standing to judge because one is intimately tied to the other person. In fact, one might be morally obligated to interfere given the social dimension of self-knowledge (see chapter 4); we deprive people we are close to of the ability to gain self-knowledge if we never comment on bad decisions they make for themselves.

Emphasizing that morality has something to say about how we treat ourselves, and that people should intervene if they have the appropriate standing when we treat ourselves badly is particularly important in the context of infertility treatment (as well as other areas of reproductive medicine). Whereas many woman stop treatment when it becomes overwhelming, some have difficulty knowing when or even how to do so. The latter was the case for Paulette Bates Alden. While in infertility treatment, she was obsessed with becoming pregnant, but since she was not having much success she knew that eventually she was going to have to quit. "I even wanted to quit. But I didn't know how. Did I have to be dead to quit? Sometimes I felt that if allowed, I would just keep on and on, never accepting it as long as I lived. I had seen a headline in the *National Enquirer* one day in the grocery line, '101-Year-Old Woman Gives Birth.' My immediate thought was that she must have been in infertility treatment and just kept on until she finally succeeded" (Alden 107). If Alden truly did not know how to quit, someone should have prevented her from continuing, not simply on the grounds that she had diminished autonomy, but that she was putting herself at serious risk of emotional and possibly even physical harm. Her behavior seriously threatened her well-being, and someone should have told her that. But, whoever that person was had to have the standing to say with authority that Alden had lost control and that she needed help putting an end to it. Most physicians do not have such standing in relation to patients.

One might state that in Alden's case it is clear that moral implications were involved in whether she stayed in treatment. But that is not necessarily true with other sorts of choices, those one might assume to be purely personal meaning that they do not entail responsibility for doing the right or the wrong thing. That is ordinarily the case with deciding to try on a pair of pants at the mall, for example, or to have potatoes instead of rice with dinner. Are we not "personally autonomous," rather than "morally autonomous," in making those kinds of choices? However, surely the question of whether I am *autonomous* in choosing potatoes or in trying on a pair of pants is out of place. It is odd to speak of autonomy in such contexts because of where the value of autonomy lies—namely, in its emancipatory potential and in the fact that people who are autonomous follow plans that give their lives purpose. If that is why autonomy is meaningful, the word should be reserved for nontrivial decisions, for those that will likely have a significant impact on the direction our lives take. A perfect example is the decision of whether to undergo infertility treatment.

Meyers did reserve discussion about autonomy for nontrivial matters, but she did not acknowledge that such decisions can have implications for whether we fulfil moral responsibilities to ourselves. Such implications arise for all autonomous and nonautonomous behaviors, which is why it is appropriate that the self-regarding attitude motivating us to be autonomous is a moral attitude. In choosing and acting autonomously, we strive to meet moral responsibilities to ourselves and possibly to others, and our will to act so stems from our trust in ourselves.

Note an important implication for bioethics of my view that purely personal decisions are irrelevant to autonomy. If autonomy and personal preference are distinct, the duty physicians have to respect our personal preferences is separate from their duty to respect our autonomy. They or anyone else can coerce us in the realm of the purely personal. For example, a physician could intimidate us into deciding to wait another half an hour for our appointment, rather than go home, which is what we prefer to do. If the decision to stay is personal, the physician has not violated our autonomy, although she may have violated her duty to respect our preferences.

The Value of Justified Self-Trust and Self-Distrust

Self-trust is therefore crucial for motivating us to be autonomous. However, not every kind of self-trust is conducive to choosing and acting autonomously precisely because autonomy has some substantive restrictions. If we trust ourselves to choose well among various options, but our beliefs about the nature of those options are inaccurate, our self-trust will actually lower our autonomy. Furthermore, if we trust ourselves without sufficient self-understanding or self-knowledge, our autonomy will suffer. Hitherto philosophers have tied the importance of self-knowledge to the idea that autonomy is about self-direction and self-discovery (Mackenzie 2000, 139, 140; Meyers 2000, 152). I link the value of self-knowledge with self-direction as well as with acknowledging one's worth as a moral agent. Those arguments establish that autonomous agents require *justified* self-trust as well as justified self-distrust.

We require self-knowledge for autonomy in part because we would not be self-directed otherwise. Following Young and Meyers, I claim that to be self-directed we must decide and act in accordance with a life plan. Now one could be guided by such a plan, yet be profoundly mistaken about whether most of one's decisions or actions conform to it; that is, about whether they are likely to advance the plan. But if one were so wrong about the likely consequences of one's actions, would we still say that one is self-directed? Consider an analogy. Would it be accurate to say that I am directing my canoe through a maze of rocks if my canoe were swerving all over and bashing into the rocks? I would have to maneuver the canoe *around* the rocks to direct it through the maze, would I not? If I were swerving all over, one would say that I was not successful in directing the canoe, or that the canoe lacked direction. The term "direction" implies some actual movement toward a goal, as opposed to utter chaos. People who are never able to actualize their life plans are not directed toward anything; they are best described as lost.

Furthermore, people should not be described as *self*-directed unless they cause their lives to move in the direction of certain goals. A person of substantial privilege might succeed in achieving his life goals with a lot of help from others, but lack self-direction if most of his success is due to his privilege. If my canoe moves smoothly through the rocks only because strong currents take it through, then *I* am not directing the canoe. Privileged people who use few of their abilities to reach their goals are only minimally self-directed. (Still, if they receive help from others only in developing their autonomy skills and in having the opportunity to exercise them, then they could be optimally self-directed.)

Self-direction, as I define it, requires self-knowledge at all three of the levels of autonomy decision making. Because direction implies movement toward a goal, it is important to be realistic when choosing how to meet our goals. And for our choices to be realistic, they have to reflect knowledge of where our competencies lie. Furthermore, our expectations about whether we will act on our choices must be realistic; they must be grounded in knowledge of how committed we are to our goals and whether we are competent to act on the decisions we have made. Finally, our judgments about whether our goals have been set by us rather than by others should be informed by knowledge of the accuracy of our judgments about the origins of our life plan. We lack such knowledge if we are in the habit of affirming "cover stories" about how our goals developed (Christman 1990, 17, cited in Stoljar 2000, 102).

Of course, to be self-directed or autonomous we do not have to be completely accurate all of the time about how competent and committed we are to succeed with our life plan. Most of us have bad days when we make bad decisions that put us behind in meeting our goals. We do not then all of a sudden become nonautonomous. Assessments of our autonomy should refer to our behavior over a significant length of time, rather than a single time at which we might have failed to exercise our autonomy. Granted, a single nonautonomous act that has enormous consequences can have a huge impact on our autonomy. Consider a woman who, like Lee, enters a fertility clinic not knowing that patients are denied access to a primary care provider and are often objectified in harmful ways as a result. The woman's decision to enter the clinic is not fully autonomous because she lacks crucial information about what she can expect there. Her autonomy will suffer because of that choice if the consequences are severe (which they were for Lee, who developed posttraumatic stress disorder). A single act of nonautonomy can destroy our autonomy, at least temporarily. Nonetheless, we can usually act nonautonomously every once in a while and still maintain our autonomy.

People can also be autonomous to varying degrees. Meyers (1989) distinguished among minimally, medially, and fully autonomous agents based on the degree to which they possess the full repertoire of autonomy skills. Roughly, a minimally autonomous agent is someone who "possesses at least some disposition to consult his or her self and at least some ability to act on his or her own beliefs, desires, and so forth" (Meyers 1989, 170). Nonetheless, that person's autonomy skills are poorly developed. Fully autonomous agents, on the other hand, are well skilled in choosing and acting autonomously, whereas the skill of medially autonomous agents lies somewhere in between those extremes. Essentially, the degree of self-knowledge that is required depends on what level of autonomy we are talking about. Autonomous agents have to have as much self-knowledge as their level of skill demands and as is required to trust themselves in a justified way to exercise (minimal, medial, or full) autonomy.

Self-knowledge is also important because of the substantive conditions for autonomy of self-worth and self-respect. To know whether we are deserving of respect or whether we possess moral worth, we must have self-knowledge. A person who does not know whether she is responsible for many of her accomplishments does not know whether to respect herself; if she does not know whether she inherently possesses moral worth, she lacks a sense of self-worth. Hence, she could not be autonomous because self-worth and self-respect are essential for autonomy.

If what we presume to know about ourselves reflects how competent and deserving we are only according to oppressive social norms, it is unlikely that we will develop self-respect or self-worth. Self-appreciative attitudes are hard to come by if negative social stereotypes define our identity. To be self-appreciative in oppressive social conditions, one has to be fairly successful screening out distorting oppressive influences. However, achieving such success is extremely difficult without at least some informational resources at hand that can expose the falsity of cultural assumptions perpetuating one's oppression. Self-knowledge is social because it flourishes in conditions in which reliable external resources can confirm or disconfirm the accuracy of one's judgments about one's self. Resources deemed reliable, or unreliable must be assessed in terms of how often they target one's actual competencies, rather than the (in)competencies one supposedly possesses according to oppressive stereotypes. Unfortunately, some people's actual competencies conform to those stereotypes because of oppressive socialization.

Thus, self-knowledge, defined against the background of a social world that is a mirror of our true selves, is essential for autonomy. It explains why self-trust motivating us to be autonomous must be justified most of the time, and also why self-distrust that is justified is often necessary. The self-trust willing us to be autonomous does not have to be well grounded—autonomy does not demand perfect self-knowledge—and neither does it have to be justified all of the time—people who are autonomous can have lazy days when they make ill-considered decisions. We only need self-trust that is *usually reliable* in targeting our true competency and commitment to stand up for our needs and values. Furthermore, we have to be able to distrust ourselves well. People who have only marginal competence in some areas because of oppressive socialization jeopardize whatever autonomy they have acquired by trusting themselves badly.[19]

Whereas self-trust of a justified sort is valuable for autonomy, the opposite is true because of the role of epistemic autonomy in the processes that make self-trust justified (see chapter 5). A reciprocal or symbiotic relation between self-trust and autonomy is possible since relations are often symbiotic (e.g., among some organisms that share ecosystems). There is no reason to assume that symbiosis could not occur among different attitudes or states of persons.

Since Lehrer shares my view that autonomy is important for self-trust, let me end this chapter by distinguishing my view of autonomy from Lehrer's. In short, I have a relational conception in which autonomy is not simply about controlling whatever influences our choices, whereas Lehrer has the opposite sort of conception.

What Susan Wolf wrote about responsibility and freedom is true of autonomy in my view: "not all things necessary for freedom and responsibility must be types of power and control. We may need simply *to be a certain way,* even though it is not within our power to determine whether we are that way or not" (Wolf 1989, 144; my emphasis). The way that we must be is "sane," which means that we have the ability "cognitively and normatively [to] recognize and appreciate the world for what it is" (Wolf 1989, 145). In other words, we must be able to distinguish between right and wrong and to perceive other aspects of the world clearly. I contend that for autonomy, we must be able "cognitively and normatively [to] recognize and appreciate" ourselves for what we are, at least to a minimal extent. We also must manifest that ability. (For Wolf, freedom and responsibility do not require that we actually use the ability she associates with sanity.)

Purely procedural theories of autonomy are about control, not about being a certain way. Lehrer endorses such a theory using the language of preferences to describe the higher-order evaluation of our desires. To be autonomous, we have to be the "author" of our preferences (Lehrer 1997, 100, 101). And that in itself is guaranteed, supposedly, if we have what he called a "power preference," namely, a preference to have the preference structure that we have. It appears that gaining the power preference is a purely procedural matter for Lehrer. It is also a purely introspective and individual matter. Alternatively, in my theory, the procedures we must follow to be autonomous are social. Autonomy *is* partly procedural is my view; it is not only about being in a certain way—namely, being someone whose mental attitudes accurately represent her own competencies and worth—for it is possible to be a certain way without being autonomous. Someone who acquires true beliefs about herself only through deference to a benevolent friend who tells her what to think about herself is hardly the perfect image of autonomy. People with autonomy must evaluate feedback they get from admired and benevolent friends. However, without such feedback, they would have trouble achieving justified attitudes of self-trust. My theory is profoundly relational, for it says that autonomous agents require a supportive social environment not only to acquire autonomy skills, but to exercise the specific skills that lead to self-knowledge and justified self-trust.

Conclusion

An environment is maximally supportive if the social forces that influence people's choices allow them to have accurate beliefs about themselves. Minimally, those forces must be nonoppressive. My discussion of problems with infertility treatment shows how oppressive social forces can inhibit self-trust at the various levels of autonomous decision making. They can interfere by confusing patients about whether they are truly competent and whether they can rely on themselves to be committed to choosing and acting autonomously. In other words, oppression can prevent patients from knowing themselves, or at least from assuming that they know themselves well enough to be able to trust themselves. For example, stereotypes about women's diminished autonomy can make some women uncertain about whether they are truly competent to make the kinds of difficult choices that often arise in infertility treatment. Double-binds, rooted in oppression, can cause profound confusion at the level of their commitment to act on one choice or another, or about their competence to judge what is motivating them to choose one way or the other.

Overall, lacking self-knowledge or simply experiencing self-doubt is a barrier to developing the kind of self-trust necessary for autonomy. It can also inhibit our autonomy if we trust ourselves to choose and act in the absence of self-knowledge. We have to get things right when trusting and distrusting ourselves because of the importance of self-knowledge and self-direction for autonomy.

The substantive and relational view of autonomy that underlies my theory of the relations between self-trust and autonomy and self-distrust and autonomy is more detailed than the standard views in bioethics. The detail is practical as well as theoretical in terms of what the theory implies for how health care providers should interpret their duty to respect the autonomy of patients. The implications demand greater respect overall for the reproductive autonomy of patients in reproductive medicine. I now turn to the practical side of the theory.

7

Improving Respect for Patient Autonomy: Patient Self-Trust in Woman-Centered Obstetrics

In reproductive medicine, gender socialization of women and dynamics of gendered and often class-based epistemic power in many patient-physician relationships are potential obstacles to patients' justified self-trust. So far we have considered the impact of gender socialization on women's ability to trust themselves well in the contexts of both miscarriage and infertility treatment. Pronatalist norms can explain why some women who have miscarried and some who have trouble deciding whether to continue with infertility treatment are self-distrustful. The epistemic authority of physicians is also a potential barrier to patient self-trust, as we saw explicitly in chapter 3 (recall Janet). At times physicians maintain such authority because patients fear that if they disagree or if they are noncompliant they will lose the support of care providers.

In bioethics and in medicine, health care providers are told that they have a duty to respect the autonomy of patients, although that is often reduced to the duty to obtain informed consent. Health care providers are rarely told to respect and promote the trust of patients in their ability to further their own goals and values, and to determine what those goals and values should be.[1] In this chapter, I use cases involving prenatal diagnosis to illustrate what health care providers can do to preserve or bolster patient self-trust. I argue that we should reconceive the duty to respect patient autonomy so that we take into account how oppression can interfere with the ability of patients to trust and distrust themselves well, and so that we acknowledge the importance of certain forms of self-trust and self-distrust for autonomy.

It is not enough, however, to argue that individual health care providers should create an optimal environment for the development and expression of patient self-trust. In many ways, the whole paradigm of medicine and the epistemology that underlies it are opposed to such an environment. Hence, we can only incorporate insights about the relation between patient self-trust and autonomy into medical practice by first making substantial changes to that practice. For example, physicians can no longer be the sole authorities on the nature and meaning of patients' bodily experiences. To have self-trust, patients must be able to define those experiences in ways with which they identify, or in ways that are integrated with their own beliefs and values. For such a change to occur in obstetrics, the field would have to become more woman (patient)-centred. In situations involving prenatal diagnosis in particular, woman-centred obstetrics would demand respect for the embodied relation of a woman to her fetus as well as for her embodied knowledge of her pregnancy.

Informed Consent, or Choice, in Theory and in Practice

Informed consent is meant to be a mechanism for preserving patient autonomy. However, because of how it is often obtained in practice, it is not a way for many patients to become autonomous agents in choosing treatments. Some bioethicists have recommended changes so that the procedure is more conducive to the exercise of patient autonomy (Lidz et al. 1988; Beauchamp and Childress 1994). Yet the recommendations of nonfeminists, in particular, fall short of identifying how power imbalances in patient-physician relationships together with cultural norms and stereotypes can interfere with patient autonomy. In the previous chapter I directed that same criticism to theories of autonomy in bioethics; now I extend it to the theory and practice of informed consent.

Normally in medical practice, informed consent occurs as a discrete event where physicians fulfil their legal obligation to disclose to patients whatever a reasonable person would want to know about the harms and benefits of a recommended procedure. After analyzing information obtained through a patient interview, physical examination, and possibly laboratory tests, the physician will inform the patient of a diagnosis or a recommended course of action, highlighting the legally relevant harms and benefits (Smith 1996, 187–190). The physician will then ask whether the patient understands and agrees with the recommended procedure and will sometimes have the patient sign a consent form. In situations where physicians are not meant to give recommendations, the physician might simply say to the patient that she has to choose based on her beliefs and values.[2] Rarely does significant communication about the patient's options occur beyond that point. Studies show that "patient-initiated questions are often 'dispreferred'" in medical interviews; yet even when patients do ask questions, they rarely challenge the accuracy of the information provided or the recommended course of action (if a recommendation is given; Smith 1996, 190).

Most patients do not question what physicians advise because of the authoritative knowledge of physicians in the area of human health. That is true for patients who welcome that authority and, ultimately, for those who oppose it. For many people who fall into the former category, what it means for them to trust their physicians is that they do not have to worry about the best approach to their care or how accurate the physician's diagnoses may be. They can simply take the physician's word for it. At the other extreme are patients for whom the knowledge of physicians is not authoritative at all. In their minds, medical knowledge may have no greater value than their own knowledge of their bodies or knowledge of alternative forms of medicine. And yet those patients may have no choice but to see a physician, and they may refrain from questioning the physician's authority for fear of being abandoned—that is, if alternative healing practices are either unavailable or are financially prohibitive. Since they tend to be in such a position because of the epistemic hegemony of medicine (which usually ensures that alternative practices are not subsidized), that hegemony underlies their reluctance to challenge their physician's authority.

American women seeking prenatal care tend to fall somewhere in between those extremes (Browner and Press 1997).[3] In other words, some advice from physicians is authoritative for them and some is not. They may reject advice about how their lifestyles should change because it is too difficult to follow given their daily routines and responsibilities. Alternatively, they reject advice because they suspect it is unfounded. What often guides them in making such decisions is their embodied knowledge derived from their perception of their pregnant body and of changes to their body that occur as pregnancy progresses (Browner and Press 1997,

113). If medical advice conflicts with that knowledge, women will often question the advice. The exception is a recommendation that is supported by medical technology, or that concerns the use of such technology (e.g., ultrasound imaging or prenatal genetic testing), in which case women are unlikely to reject it. It seems that what really is authoritative for many women in prenatal health care in the United States is medical technology, not physicians (Browner and Press 1997).

Yet for some of those women, one might question whether the technology is even authoritative. An alternative explanation for why some women consent to ART is that they believe they have little opportunity to refuse. The difference between advice about lifestyle changes and about having, say, an ultrasound is that women can dismiss the former, but usually not the latter without the physician finding out about it. They can listen to advice about lifestyle changes, knowing full well that they will not follow it. They cannot do the same with an ultrasound.

Browner and Press (1997) did not find that when pregnant women reject medical advice they do so openly with their physicians. Thus, prenatal visits might still conform to the pattern I described for patient-physician interviews. Whereas many women probably do prefer technological monitoring of pregnancy and birth, the dynamics of the relationship that some women have with physicians make it difficult for them ever to refuse what the physician recommends.

Many bioethicists oppose the traditional dynamic of patient-physician interviews and the way that informed consent is often obtained in them. When patients consent to procedures that physicians recommend, there is no guarantee that the decision will be right for them, given *their* values, life goals, and social circumstances (Lidz et al. 1988). Patients are not autonomous unless they participate in a meaningful way in the decision-making process. Of course, they also must have the opportunity to refuse as well as to consent; that is, they must be able to make a choice. Baylis proposed a shift toward the language of "informed choice" (1993, ftn 1) that is not merely semantic, but reflects an enlightened view of the nature of autonomous decision making.

Some bioethicists claim that to satisfy the conditions for autonomy, informed choice should occur as an interactive process, rather than as a single event at which physicians disclose information (Lidz et al. 1988;

Beauchamp and Childress 1994). As I discussed in chapter 5, the following is the standard list of conditions for autonomy in contemporary bioethics: patients must be competent, or have decisional capacity; they must possess the relevant understanding; and they must choose and act voluntarily. To ensure the presence of each of these conditions, advocates of the "process model" of informed choice hold that physicians have to engage with patients in evaluating available options, and assist patients in making decisions that are consistent with the latters' values. Through active involvement of patients in negotiating the approach to care, physicians should be able to learn whether patients have decisional capacity,[4] and of whether they are likely to choose freely rather than under the influence of some coercive or manipulative force.

Furthermore, giving patients the opportunity to ask questions and to express concerns should improve their understanding of the relevant medical information. Only once patients appreciate the significance of that information for their own lives—meaning that they are aware of possible or probable changes that could occur in their lives if they were to choose any of the options—is the condition for autonomy of understanding satisfied (Appelbaum and Roth 1982). Moreover, to achieve such a level of awareness, patients have to factor in nonmedical information about the possible or probable impact of a particular decision on their work, for example, on their sense of themselves, or on their relationships with others.

To be in a position to help patients understand their options in the relevant way, it is crucial that physicians develop relationships with them. One of the ethical problems in the case of Lee (see Introduction) is that she was denied such a relationship. She was the victim of a disturbing trend in Canadian medicine (and perhaps in other health care systems as well) toward a team approach to treatment that provides no guarantee of a primary care provider.[5] Patients are shuffled among physicians, making it highly unlikely that physicians will know patients well enough to have a sense of the significance of different options for their lives.

Advocates of the process model also recommend that physicians clarify their values and expectations so that patients can understand why physicians recommend a particular treatment (Lidz et al. 1988, 1386). Although I do not think that revealing one's values to patients is always appropriate (as I discuss below), I agree with a point underlying that recommendation: that physicians must realize that their advice is not value free. It presupposes values, which in reproductive contexts often include the value of having a "perfect baby," or overcoming infertility even at a substantial personal cost. Patients *can* disagree with their physicians about which value assumptions should guide the approach to their care.

The process model of informed choice does identify many of the problems with the standard "event model"; however, it does not go far enough in addressing potential barriers to autonomy in interactions between patients and physicians. If physicians were open and honest about their values and expectations, that might diffuse some of their epistemic power, thereby leaving more room for patient involvement in decision making. But as we have seen, physicians gain at least some of that power through the technology they use to support their diagnoses. For many of us, the authority of medical technology goes unquestioned (Davis-Floyd 1992; Browner and Press 1997); however, not all of it warrants the exalted status we give it. A prime example is a maternal serum test, which is a form of prenatal genetic screening that has a false positive rate of approximately 5%, increasing to over 40% for women over the age of 35 (Mennuti 1996, 1442). The test assesses a woman's blood for serum markers that are predictive of Down syndrome and of open neural tube defects,[6] but it can only inform a woman of her individual *risk* for having a fetus with either genetic anomaly. Thus, the meaning of a positive result is ambiguous on two fronts: because of the high rate of false positives; and because the result is still only an indication of risk. In spite of the ambiguity, few women refuse the test when it is offered to them (Browner and Press 1995). And although a variety of factors may influence such a decision (as I illustrate below), a prominent factor surely is the power of medical technology.

Missing from most process accounts of informed choice is acknowledgment not only of how norms about technology can interfere with patient autonomy, but of how oppression can have the same effect. They tend to leave out the important condition for autonomy that the formation of our self-concept, values, and goals should be authentic rather than influenced by coercive forces, including forces of oppression. Although such forces are not necessarily directed toward or away from one of the patient's options (see chapter 6), advocates of the process model usually assume that coercion must have that focus. Oppressive stereotypes can lower the self-appreciation of some patients, and their threat is often heightened in interactions with physicians, most of whom are members of dominant groups. Oppressive norms may have the overall effect of inhibiting some patients from participating in the decision making process at all. It is not enough to recommend that all patients be encouraged to participate because the reasons some do not are more complex than absence of encouragement. Some patients lack self-trust, which means either that they will not be inclined to participate or they will participate only in such a way that they defer ultimately to the judgment of the physician.

In the previous chapter I identified many obstacles to the formation of justified attitudes of self-trust for patients who are oppressed, and I highlight a few others in this chapter. However, my main purpose here is to suggest how physicians can minimize those barriers, and how the practice of medicine can be conceived differently to allow for the preservation or promotion of patient self-trust. My discussion centres on obstetrics, although many recommendations I make are relevant to other areas of medicine. Furthermore, by focusing on obstetrics, my aim is not to reinforce the hegemony of physicians caring for pregnant women. I accept that midwives and doulas might be better than physicians at encouraging patients to trust themselves. I also recommend that obstetrical care be more interdisciplinary than it currently tends to be, so that social workers, for example, and other types of counselors play a more integral role.

Promoting Self-Trust About Prenatal Diagnosis: The Level of Choice

There are three levels of autonomous decision making: choosing well, acting on our choices, and judging the authenticity of the values and goals that inform our choices. My theory of autonomy is more elaborate in many ways than the standard theory in contemporary bioethics; for example, at the level of choosing well, we require more than just decisional capacity and understanding. We have to be able to identify with first-order attitudes that influence our choices and have justified trust in our ability to choose well. Such justification is contingent on whether the source of the information we use to understand our situation is reliable, and on whether we have knowledge of the accuracy of our decision-making skills and of our competence and commitment to do what our decision required of us (if anything). Self-knowledge is a substantive condition for autonomy, which is why the self-trust motivating us to choose autonomously must be justified.

The following case illustrates many of the potential obstacles to justified self-trust in patients at the level of choosing well in the context of prenatal genetic testing. It is based on observations I made in prenatal clinics and genetic counseling sessions while doing a clinical practicum in ethics and obstetrics at a maternity and children's hospital. The case is also consistent with sociological and anthropological literature on the pressures many women feel in Western culture when deciding whether to undergo prenatal genetic testing.

Lara is a 37-year-old woman, pregnant for the first time. She and her partner, Frank, had been trying to conceive for years and were only now successful. Lara has worked hard at her career and knows she will have to cut back on her workload once the baby is born. Frank, on the other hand, will continue to work full-throttle to promote his thriving new business. He does not feel that he can take time off even to accompany Lara to prenatal visits.[7]

At her first visit, Lara asks the obstetrician about prenatal diagnosis. Her obstetrician informs her that the generic risk for a person of her age for having a child with down syndrome is 1 in 227 (0.4%) and that the total risk for chromosomal abnormalities is 1 in 130 (0.8%). Lara's options are as follows: chorionic villus sampling, which is a diagnostic test done at 10 to 11 weeks' gestation and carries a 1% to 1.5% risk of pregnancy loss; amniocentesis at 16 to 17 weeks, which is also diagnostic and has a 0.5% loss rate; and maternal serum screening at 16 to 17 weeks, which will not diagnose a fetal abnormality, but will tell Lara her individual risk for having a child with Down syndrome or an open neural tube defect. If that test is positive, Lara can elect to have a detailed ultrasound or amniocentesis. Depending on the timing of the screening test, she would receive the results of amniocentesis at approximately 19 to 20 weeks' gestation.[8]

Lara brings that information home to Frank so that they can determine together what the risk of having a child with a disability means to them and what the risks of the procedures mean as well. Lara soon learns that Frank does not give much weight to the issue of whether she has prenatal testing.[9] He assumes that the risk of having a child with a disability is so low that they really should not worry about it. Still, he says that if a genetic screen or test is common, particularly for women of Lara's age, she might as well have it done.

For Lara, the decision is hardly that straightforward. She is concerned about the risk of having a child with a disability, as she fears that she would not be able to care properly for such a child (knowing that she would be the child's primary caregiver). Intellectually, she is not opposed to abortion, yet emotionally it is difficult for her even to imagine terminating this pregnancy since she has longed to have a child for years. Hence, the loss rates of the diagnostic procedures worry her considerably. Lara is also concerned that a choice she makes could elicit negative responses from people she respects.[10] For example, if she decides to forego the diagnostic tests, some would regard her as irresponsible. If the results of amniocentesis done after serum screening convince her that she should terminate her pregnancy after twenty weeks, some would wonder if she had any maternal instincts at all.

The complexity of her options and the conflicts among her concerns and desires leave her profoundly confused. She is frustrated with Frank because he persists in denying what she perceives to be a serious issue. Lara desperately wants to make the right decision, but she is not sure that she is capable of determining what that is on her own.

Lara is in a classic double-bind, one that originates partly in the mixed messages she has received from society about prenatal genetic testing. If she refuses testing, she is irresponsible, since a strong voice in her community assumes it is irresponsible to bring a child with a disability into the world. And it may actually be irresponsible if it is true that she could not care properly for such a child. Consenting to testing, on the other hand, could place her on a path toward a second-trimester abortion, which is a heartless act for any mother, according to the dictates of a different segment of her community. It would also be an extremely difficult act for Lara because of her history of infertility.

Lara distrusts herself to choose well because of the double-bind, because of the complexity of her options, and because she feels that she lacks support from people close to her (namely, Frank) for making the right decision. Her options are complex because of the small risks they entail for her and for her potential future child, and because of the conflicts between her values and goals in that domain. Interpreting risks involves making value judgments, for what a risk means, however small, depends on how much we devalue whatever we put ourselves at risk for. Lara is confused about what a 0.4% risk for Down syndrome means for her perhaps because the risk is so small, but also because she does not know how much she should devalue having a child with a disability (compared with possibly having no child at all). She would not necessarily be in a better position to choose well even if her risk for having a child with Down syndrome were to increase significantly, say to 4.4%. Thus the option of discovering what her individual risk is through maternal serum screening may not appeal to her.

That Frank does not share or perhaps even comprehend Lara's concerns contributes to her self-distrust. She feels that she needs help from others in deciding what to do, and she thought that some would be forthcoming from Frank, with whom she has probably sorted through difficult decisions in the past. Her self-distrust is profoundly relational (in the sense of being socially constituted), where the relevant relations are those with Frank and with people in her community whom she respects but whose views contradict one another.

Another factor that will shape whether Lara trusts herself to choose well is her relationship with the obstetrician. Individual obstetricians can be expected neither to free women from the double-binds of prenatal genetic testing nor to eliminate the difficulty of deciding in the face of small risks. However, they can try to ensure that women and their partners have whatever support, time, and information they require to sort through their decision.

Lara's obstetrician could help her to determine which side of the double-bind she may find the most persuasive in the end. It would be inappropriate, though, for the obstetrician to reveal which side *she* finds the most persuasive. Health care providers should show equal support from their perspective for authorizing testing or for refusing it, as well for termination or continuation of a pregnancy if a patient learns that her fetus has a genetic abnormality.[11] Contrary to the recommendation of some advocates of the process model, it is not always appropriate for physicians to reveal their values to patients. In the context of prenatal diagnosis, they should refrain from adding to the pressure that many women feel "to be responsible" and to have tests done.[12] A strong connection in North America already exists between maternal responsibility and prenatal diagnosis (Mitchell and Georges 1998, 118; Charo and Rothenberg 1994), (although as Lara's case illustrates, that connection is riddled with inconsistencies. Conventional wisdom has it that "good mothers" do not risk giving birth to a child with a disability (Charo and Rothenberg 1994), but how good could they be as mothers if they could terminate a pregnancy in the second trimester?)

It is questionable whether some women *autonomously* accept the responsibility of having prenatal testing. They may have values that conflict with that view of their maternal obligations and with that degree of medical intervention in their pregnancies. Not all women or men are adverse to having a child with a disability, and that is especially true of parents who already have such a child (Wertz et al. 1991, cited in Charo and Rothenberg 1994, 106). Others simply do not want to be placed in the position of having to choose "the kind of baby [they]'d get" (Rapp 1997, 138). White middle-class women, in particular, tend to be ambivalent toward prenatal diagnosis (Rapp 1997). While they might view the technology as authoritative (Browner and Press 1997), they also believe that with that kind of medical intervention they have less control over their pregnancies than they otherwise would (Rapp 1997, 139). In consenting to testing they may simply be complying with the societal view that technological monitoring of pregnancy is necessary. They might not be choosing autonomously. That does not mean that rejecting testing altogether would be an autonomous choice for many women either. Some women feel that they have little alternative but to undergo testing because raising a child with a disability is not an option given their social and financial circumstances. Still, they might agree that it is not necessarily any woman's maternal responsibility to have prenatal genetic tests.

Critics would conclude that whereas social pressure to have prenatal tests might restrict the reproductive freedom of some women, the limit is justified because of (what they see as) the suffering and financial burden on society that accompanies the birth of a child with a disability. If women are morally obligated to have these tests, obstetricians and other clinicians *should* encourage them to have it, rather than support the options of authorization and refusal equally. However, that view is highly contentious for a number of reasons. One is that rarely do diagnostic tests for fetal abnormalities reveal the degree of suffering that a child with a disability will experience. A positive test result for many conditions, including Down syndrome, neural tube defects, and sickle cell anemia, indicates only the presence of the abnormality, not its severity.[13] But even if the tests could be more informative, only a small percentage of disabilities are genetic anyway. And if it is in society's interest to prevent disability, which it may well not be,[14] before violating women's reproductive freedom, we should strive to prevent forms of disability that are not genetic (e.g. by improving road safety or the safety of workplace environments; Charo and Rothenberg 1994).

If prenatal testing is merely permissible, not obligatory morally speaking, counseling for it should be nondirective. Moreover, the counseling may have to come from professionals who are better equipped than physicians to assist patients in loosening the double-binds of prenatal diagnosis, with the aim of enhancing patient self-trust. Patients have to develop self-trust in a way that is justified and that therefore reflects self-knowledge concerning their ability to make a decision that is consistent with their goals and values, and that is realistic given their competencies and commitments. Furthermore, to know what is realistic, they have to have adequate understanding of their options. Lara seems to assume that her life would be altered in mostly negative ways if she were to give birth to a child with a disability. Yet before she can know that with any certainty, she must find out what disabling conditions of different genetic disorders are and what social services would be available to her if she were to have a child with one of those disorders. She should be able to seek counseling from a social worker who could outline the available social services, and from a genetic counselor or who could describe the nature of different genetic disorders and possibly put her in touch with parents who have raised children with those disorders.

Some would claim that proliferating discussion about a woman's decision of whether to have prenatal testing by ensuring that the kind of counseling I recommended be available would simply increase the "tentativeness" of modern pregnancies. As a result of prenatal diagnosis, women are forced into "tentative pregnancies," where they hesitate to feel good about their pregnancies until the test results are back (Rothman 1986). This view implies that to allow women to have positive pregnancy experiences, we should not offer them prenatal testing. However, it is not clear that eliminating testing is a good idea, especially in our ableist and sexist society where social assistance is poor for people with disabilities as well as for people who care for them, most of whom are women (Kittay 1999). Abolishing testing would also be problematic for women who have fetuses with horrendous abnormalities (e.g., anencephaly), and who would want to be spared the shock and emotional pain of giving birth to the child. Still, if women are to have the option of prenatal screening and diagnosis, it is important that all of the necessary information is available, including possible and probable changes to their lives if they had a child with a certain disability. Only then could they develop *justified* attitudes of self-trust toward their decision.

Also relevant to decisions about prenatal testing is information about follow-up care that patients could expect on choosing each option. Women such as Lara have to know whether, where, and for how long abortion services would be available if they were to receive a positive test result and decide in favor of terminating the pregnancy. If they were to choose prenatal testing in the absence of such knowledge and had the goal of not having a child with a disability, the choice would not necessarily enhance their self-direction. They might not have the option of having a second-trimester abortion, since in Canada and the United States, at least, they have no legal right to such services. Whether they have that option in Canada usually depends on how far along they are in the second trimester. Restrictions on when second-trimester abortions can be performed are dictated by hospital policy, which tends to vary from one province to the next.[15]

From the point of view of promoting patient self-trust, women and their partners should have the necessary time to sort through whatever complex array of factors is influencing their choice of whether to have prenatal testing and whether to terminate a pregnancy when faced with a positive diagnosis. Providing that time by loosening restrictions on second-trimester terminations is not an ideal solution because of how emotionally wrenching those abortions can be. Still, current time pressures on couples to decide about prenatal diagnosis and a possible termination are inappropriate. If a woman has a positive serum screen, for example, usually she and her partner are forced to decide about further testing *during* an appointment for genetic counseling, where they learn the results of the test and are given information about the disorder. Often, a tentative appointment is made for a diagnostic procedure immediately after the counseling session because the window of opportunity for further testing and for possible termination is so small, given restrictions on terminations (Charo and Rothenberg 1994, 109). Clearly, that gives women, or couples, very little time to absorb information and to weigh all of the relevant factors. Counseling must be given earlier in the pregnancies of women who opt for testing, at which point they and their partners should be encouraged to reflect on the information they receive, rather than be forced to consider it all of a sudden on receiving test results.

Of course, more time and more information with which to decide about prenatal testing cannot ensure that patients will trust themselves in a justified way to choose well. Yet even if they cannot develop that self-trust, physicians do not necessarily have the moral authority to decide on their behalf. Even if Lara were given ample time and information, she might persist in distrusting herself to make the right decision. And her distrust would be understandable because the decision is inherently difficult given the small risks she has to weigh and the complicated social factors she must take into account. However, the obstetrician is in no better position than she is to make that decision because of its inherent difficulty. In fact, the obstetrician is probably in a worse position because she knows less than Lara about Lara's values and social circumstances. Therefore, she should not intervene paternalistically. Such a response would be unwarranted even if Lara were 47 instead of 37 (and so had a higher risk for Down syndrome) and had a family history of a congenital abnormality. In that case, even if the obstetrician felt strongly that Lara should consent to some prenatal diagnosis, she should not take the decision away from her, especially since Lara has no clear obligation to accept (or refuse).

The objection against paternalism here is *not* that a paternalistic response would be disrespectful of Lara's autonomy; it is that the obstetrician cannot presume to know any better than Lara which option is best for her. It is not clear that there is any space for autonomy because of Lara's persistent and profound self-distrust. Thus, if she were to request that the obstetrician decide on her behalf, it would not violate her autonomy for the obstetrician to agree. Whether Lara defers to the obstetrician's judgment or struggles to choose from a position of profound self-distrust, she does not exercise autonomy. By deferring, she fulfils a desire to have someone else decide for her, and that is hardly even a minimally autonomous desire. Thus, if there is no room for autonomy, there can be no objection from the point of view of respecting Lara's autonomy to a consensual form of paternalism. Even so, the obstetrician should be uncomfortable with that solution, as she would have to assume at some level to know what the right decision is for Lara, which again is a problematic assumption.

Overall, self-trust as a condition for autonomy should not be viewed as a potential avenue for paternalistic intervention. Like the condition of understanding, physicians have an obligation to promote or preserve the self-trust of patients, but not to attempt to remove patients' decisional authority if they do not trust themselves (unless, of course, they clearly lack decisional capacity). Such a response is inappropriate even where the physician does understand a patient's values, goals, and social circumstances well enough to make a decision on her behalf that would truly promote her interests. If that were the case, the physician should also know how the patient should trust herself, and could encourage her to develop that trust in a way that would preserve her autonomy.

Part of the task of providing encouragement is for physicians themselves to trust patients to make decisions that are right for themselves. We can hardly expect patients to trust their competency in being autonomous if physicians distrust it. Hence, it is reasonable to suppose that physicians have an obligation to trust, or at least to cultivate trust, in patients' autonomy skills.

But whether patients will welcome the trust of physicians may depend on whether the trust is reciprocated. The distrust of patients in their own ability to choose well can persist not only because of the inherent complexity of the decision, but because they cannot rely on the information that is relevant to their choice or they cannot trust the purveyor of that information. Some women are sceptical of the accuracy of information provided by prenatal genetic testing (Rapp 1998, 155). Others are distrustful of medicine generally because of how members of their social group have been treated by medical professionals historically or even recently. Rapp describes a case of a black couple that refused amniocentesis once they discovered that the leftover amniotic fluid could be used in medical experiments (1998, 146, 147). They were informed that they could say "no" to its experimental use, but they refused nonetheless, presumably because they distrusted the technicians not to experiment with the fluid against their wishes. Their distrust could easily have stemmed from fear that results of the experiments would be harmful to black people, just as methods of performing some experiments were in the past (e.g., the Tuskegee syphilis experiment).

To bolster patient self-trust at the level of choosing well, health care providers have to gain the trust of patients and strive to overcome barriers to trust with patients who may have good reason to distrust them. To achieve those ends, they must display moral integrity and competence in addressing patients' health care needs. Acting with integrity means that they honor their commitments to patients, and if they fail to meet a specific commitment they take some responsibility for the harm or disappointment they have caused. Trust thrives only where optimism about competence and moral integrity exists. However, interpersonal trust also involves two expectations (see chapter 2): that the values of people we trust are similar to our own values in the relevant domain; and that they perceive their relationship with us similarly to the way we perceive it. To try to encourage the first expectation in patients, health care providers could clearly state what they value, in a general sense, about patient care. For example, they could assure patients that they are committed to promoting their well-being and to respecting their autonomy. Declaring such values would be beneficial, unlike announcing what their values are concerning prenatal genetic tests.

To encourage the second expectation, health care providers could assure patients that they perceive the relationship with them to be professional. In trusting, we must expect the trusted person to share our perception of our relationship because the commitments we can reasonably expect someone to fulfil differ depending on the type of relationship we have. It follows that patients can more easily trust health care providers to honor the sorts of commitments one can reasonably expect them to fulfill (depending on their specific profession) if the providers ensure that their relationships with patients remain on a professional level.

Note, also, that caution is necessary in establishing trust when health care providers know or suspect that a patient is in an abusive relationship or has a history of physical or sexual abuse. Obstetrical patients are more likely than others to experience severe abuse because the abuse of women in heterosexual relationships tends to increase in pregnancy (Stewart and Cecutti 1993). Survivors often have problems with trusting, or distrusting, because they have trusted others whom they should have been able to trust, but who betrayed them severely (Herman 1992, 51, 52). Rather than perpetuate damage to their trust skills, health care providers should not expect trust from those patients until they give patients ample evidence that they themselves are trustworthy (Lepine 1990, 275). Here is an example of what that might mean in practice: in performing a physical examination or procedure, the health care provider could ask the patient frequently if she is all right, rather than simply expect that she will be all right and will not fear being violated again.

As I stated in chapter 4, abuse and oppression can interfere with a patient's trust in her ability to make autonomous choices. She might have the ability, yet be convinced otherwise because she has internalized hateful messages from an abuser or from a racist, sexist, or classist society. Alternatively, her oppression or abuse may have starved her of necessary skills for choosing autonomously, which is why she distrusts herself in that regard. Thus, the self-distrust of a patient in Lara's situation might persist neither because of the complexity of her decision nor because she cannot rely on relevant medical information, but because she cannot or does not know how to trust herself. The tendency to defer to the judgment of others would be natural for her; but rather than reinforce it, the physician should either take the time to guide her through the decision-making process or involve a counselor in that process who could take the necessary time. By allowing the patient to defer to the physician's judgment, the physician would be perpetuating her self-distrust and risking that the care the patient receives is inconsistent with whatever goals and values the patient has that are relevant to her choice.

The potential obstacles to patient self-trust at the level of choosing well are therefore varied, and they require varied responses from health care providers. Providers could follow certain general rules nonetheless to en-hance justified self-trust in patients surrounding prenatal testing. For ex-ample, they could assure patients that they would respect either the decision to opt for testing or to refuse it. They could give patients the kind of information that would improve their knowledge of the conse-quences of choosing each option and necessary time to absorb that in-formation. Finally, they could allow patients to rely on the information by allowing them to trust its source (i.e., themselves).

The Level of Action: Combating Stereotype Threats

Barriers to patient self-trust at the level of acting on choices overlap significantly with barriers at the level of choosing well. Double-binds can interfere at both levels. They can cause women to distrust their ability to act on a decision to forego prenatal testing because of a lingering desire to avoid the censure they would receive from some members of their community. Lacking information that is relevant to how they would cope with the consequences of a particular decision can also inhibit justified self-trust in acting autonomously. Obviously, recommendations for re-moving those obstacles are the same at both levels of autonomy.

Here, I want to focus on barriers to patient self-trust that are specific to acting autonomously and that concern the power imbalance in many patient-physician relationships. An example is a stereotype threat where the patient has not internalized what the stereotype says about her, but is fearful about living up to it in the eyes of the physician. I have men-tioned the influence of stereotypes often, but have yet to give a case where a patient feels that influence without actually believing the stereotype.

Melissa is 25 years old in her second pregnancy and without a stable partner. She has very little formal education, having quit school after grade 9. At each prenatal visit the physician asks if she has any questions or concerns about her prenatal care. Melissa usually shakes her head, de-spite often having concerns. She is not normally shy, nor does she believe that her concerns about her pregnancy are trivial. She does not have a pas-sive personality, nor does she lack confidence in her own judgment. Melissa comes from a working-class family in which women learn to re-spect themselves in relation to men, but in which people who are uneducated are perceived to be fundamentally inferior to the educated. The latter are revered almost like gods. Melissa herself has always been frustrated with how her parents belittle themselves in front of people with "higher education." Their behavior has made her eminently aware of the cultural stereotype of uneducated people as intellectually inferior. Melissa assumes that her physician's view of her is influenced by that stereotype, and she does not trust herself to express her concerns to him without reinforcing the truth of that stereotype in his mind. So to be on the safe side, she decides to keep her concerns to herself.

Whenever her obstetrician recommends something to her, Melissa consents. When he offers her prenatal diagnosis and tells her it is up to her to choose whether she wants it or not, she chooses it, assuming that he must believe she should have it, since otherwise he would not offer it. Moreover, being a member of the medical profession, he must be in favor of such technologies she assumes, for whenever she met physicians in the past, they always were quick to defend any new medical development. Melissa would actually prefer not to have a prenatal test—she wants only minimal medical intervention in her pregnancy—but she does not want to risk the physician thinking that she is therefore naive or ignorant.

Melissa does not lack self-trust at the level of choosing autonomously; she trusts herself to decide what counts as a nontrivial concern about her prenatal care, for example. Furthermore, with her family and among friends she trusts herself to voice her concerns and to act on her choices. She lacks self-trust at that level of autonomy only during prenatal visits. There, she presumes that she has entered a world that constructs her differently than the world she normally inhabits. Stereotypes can infect some "worlds" but not others, to use Maria Lugones's terminology (1987), and hence, the behavior of people stereotyped can shift dramatically as they move between different worlds.

Even if people do not internalize them, stereotypes can influence behavior by preventing people from acting autonomously. I might internalize the construction of me in hostile worlds, or alternatively, "I may not accept [that construction] as an account of myself" (Lugones 1987, 10). Yet even if I reject the stereotype, I might be *animating* it in the eyes of another (Lugones 1987, 10; her emphasis). I might be giving life to it, either intentionally, perhaps as a way of revealing its absurdity,[16] or un-intentionally, because I do not have complete control over how others interpret what I do or who I am. Thus, people with "arrogant eyes" might perceive me through the lens of a stereotype even though there is little evidence of the truth of it in my behavior (Frye 1983). If Melissa is right that the physician believes in the stereotype of uneducated people, even if she were to speak articulately and to ask intelligent questions about her prenatal care, he might judge her stereotypically nonetheless. Melissa still seems to assume that she *could* control how he perceives her; she simply distrusts that ability, which in turn interferes with her autonomy.

Behavior such as Melissa's is not uncommon among people who are subject to oppressive stereotypes (Steele 1995, 1997).[17] They can feel these threats even if they do not accept the stereotypes on an unconscious level. One might be inclined to assume that unconsciously, through the influence of her family, Melissa does believe in the stereotype of uneducated people. Yet to reject her own explanation for why she behaves passively is both unnecessary and uncharitable. She is concerned about reinforcing a stereotype in *someone else's* mind, not in her own mind, as she herself claims.

However, there is one stereotype influencing Melissa's behavior that she does believe in: that physicians rarely question the value of new medical technologies. Patients often arrive at clinics with preconceptions about the value commitments of health care providers. Melissa's stereotypical view is probably common, as is the preconception that obstetricians have a strong bias in favor of creating perfect babies.

Given such stereotypes, what might amount to equal support from physicians for a patient's options surrounding prenatal genetic testing is to emphasize that they *do*, in fact, support the option of refusal. To minimize the influence of Melissa's stereotype of physicians, her physician could say that he does not expect her to choose prenatal testing. But if she did make that choice, he would not assume that she would necessarily want further testing or to terminate her pregnancy if the results were positive. Care is necessary, however, in taking such an approach. It could send the wrong message; namely, that Melissa is too stupid to understand what kind of choice situation she is in. The approach also might seem appropriate to some physicians only because, deep down, they truly believe that some patients are "too stupid." Physicians must reflect carefully on their own motives when combating stereotype threats.

To anticipate such threats in first place, health care providers should be aware of common biases and stereotypes in our culture. They then have to do whatever they can to minimize the negative effects.[18] For example, instead of being complacent with passive patients who are the target of oppressive stereotypes, they should wonder whether they are experiencing a stereotype threat. They could even work with that presumption in such cases. The perceived threat is relevant not only to patients who have little education compared with physicians, but also to female patients with male physicians, to black patients with white physicians, to patients with disabilities whose physicians are able-bodied, and so on. Such patients can easily feel anxious about seeming less capable than the professional who stands before them about making sound judgments that further their own interests.

Other recommendations for diminishing stereotype threats appear in Steele's work (1997, 624, 625). He suggests being optimistic about the person's ability to perform well or to make good decisions, and to challenge that person with difficult decisions, which shows respect for his abilities. Above, I wrote that obstetricians should display trust in patients' abilities to handle decisions around prenatal diagnosis. They could do that with passive patients, while acknowledging how complex those decisions can be. The alternative of simply removing the decision-making authority of passive patients who feel the threat of a stereotype would not only diminish the autonomy of those patients, it would probably convince them that despite active efforts to the contrary, they confirmed the stereotype about them. To prevent such an outcome, physicians also might involve other health care providers or counselors in communicating with patients. Women patients with men physicians or patients who are less educated than physicians might feel more comfortable expressing their opinions to a female doula or to a female nurse.

The position of power that physicians occupy poses a further barrier to patient self-trust that is relative to the level of acting on one's choices: the fear of losing the support of one's care provider, which stands in the way of patient's refusing the advice of a physician. Patients have to know that if they refuse physicians' recommendations they will not be abandoned, that even if conflicts arise that appear to threaten physicians' professional or personal integrity, the physicians will either attempt a compromise or will refer patients to different care providers. Either should occur unless, of course, the patient's refusal or request violates fundamental moral norms of our society (e.g., if the request is to have an abortion for the purpose of sex selection).

Aside from assurances against abandonment and against the threat of being judged stereotypically, a woman contemplating prenatal testing cannot trust herself to act on an autonomous decision if she lacks bodily integrity. If a third party is dictating whatever decisions she makes in her pregnancy, and hence usurping control over what happens to her body, she will lack self-trust at the level of acting autonomously. That is not the only level, however, at which absence of bodily integrity can interfere with self-trust. Bodily integrity is also important at the level of judging whether one truly endorses the self-concept, goals, and values reflected in one's choices.

The Level of Authenticity: Respecting Bodily Integrity

Autonomous agents must be able to trust their judgment about the authenticity of the attitudes influencing their choices, and furthermore, their self-conceptions have to be consistent with their worth, since self-worth and self-respect are substantive conditions for autonomy. How people conceive of themselves determines which goals and values they endorse and act upon. If their self-conceptions are fragmented or confused, they will probably be confused about what they truly value and desire. We saw some evidence of that in the case of Lee (see Introduction). The objectification she suffered during infertility treatment alienated her, to some degree, from the needs, desires, and values with which she would normally identify as a self-respecting person, one whose moral status is not reduced to the level of her reproductive capacity (or lack thereof). She could no longer identify with the person she once was, and that made her distrust her judgment about what she truly desired and valued.

Patients can lose trust in their own judgment without experiencing an assault on their identity as persons, however. As we saw in chapter 3 with Anna, a woman can be confused after a miscarriage about how she should value her fetus and interpret its death if others surrounding her do not give uptake to her feelings. Anna's interpretation of her miscarriage was mediated by presumed and perhaps actual comments from others about how it was "a blessing in disguise" or a relatively insignificant event compared with a stillbirth, especially since it occurred early in the first trimester. Such views were disrespectful of Anna's experience, which clearly held great personal significance for her. She could not trust her judgment about its significance, however, because her feelings contradicted what her society implied that she should feel.

Lee's self-distrust, and possibly Anna's as well, arose in part because they were denied bodily integrity, as Mackenzie interpreted that concept (1992). Bodily integrity is normally understood in terms of our ability to control what happens to our bodies (Boetzkes 1999, 121).[19] According to Mackenzie, we should extend our use of that concept to the control we have (or lack) over our perspective on our bodies, or on our own bodily experiences. Although such a perspective is always mediated by cultural and social images of bodies (we cannot expect to free ourselves of those images), we lose bodily integrity when we are persuaded to adopt bodily perspectives with which we do not identify. Lee did not identify with the idea that her body and, more specifically, her reproductive parts, are constitutive of her self. That view was reflected in the behavior of the people in the operating room who ignored her existence and denied her emotional needs. Anna self-distrust about the emotional significance of her miscarriage was probably bound up with how she perceived her bodily relation to her fetus. Whereas presumably in the minds of others that relation barely existed (the fetus was only six weeks' gestation), in her mind the fetus may have become a part of her already, which would explain why its death had such a profound affect on her.

I maintain that significant barriers exist to the kind of bodily integrity Mackenzie (1992) described for patients in modern obstetrics, particularly in contexts involving prenatal genetic testing. The resulting moral harm is that patients are less able to have self-trust, and hence autonomy, at the level of deciding which beliefs and values should influence their choices. (Below, I acknowledge that some patients can have bodily perspectives that are harmful ultimately to themselves or their fetuses and that health care providers must persuade them to alter or relinquish those perspectives.)

Women commonly feel that they do not have control over their perception of their bodies; but that feeling can intensify in pregnancy when they are subject to inner as well as outer assaults on their bodily perspectives. Pregnant women must contend with cultural images of their inner bodies, of their bodily relation to their fetus, as well as with the social myths about their outer appearance. Prenatal ultrasound has introduced into Western culture the image of the fetus as a free-floating entity, as many feminists have noted (Overall 1993, 40–41; Petchesky 1987). Pro-life activists also frequently display enhanced images of the baby-like qualities of fetuses to further their political agendas. By contrast, some pro-choice literature (particularly in philosophy) portrays the fetus as a parasitic being that threatens to deprive the woman of her freedom (Thomson 1971). Any of those constructions of the maternal-fetal dyad can conflict with the way a woman experiences pregnancy and views her relationship with her fetus. If she is barraged with any particular set of images, her bodily integrity may suffer.

In Mackenzie's definition, bodily integrity in pregnancy demands a bodily perspective that is compatible with the way a woman views not only her physical relation to her fetus, but also her moral relation to it. Bodily integrity "in pregnancy and abortion . . . is a question of being able to shape for oneself an integrated bodily perspective, a perspective by means of which a woman can respond to the bodily processes that she experiences in a way with which she identifies, and in a way that is consistent with the decision she makes concerning her future moral relationship with the foetus" (Mackenzie 1992, 151). If the woman's decision about that relationship is to end it, but she is bombarded with pro-life images of fetuses, for example, she may lose some bodily integrity. Similarly, outside of or within pregnancy, the contempt for many women's bodies that cultural images of beauty promote can conflict with a woman's conception of her moral worth. Hence, those images are potential obstacles to her bodily integrity, if such integrity has a moral element to it.

Forces that undermine our bodily integrity can generate distrust at the level of evaluating whether we are capable of being morally responsible, and if so, where our moral responsibilities lie. When women are objectified according to cultural images that are disdainful of their bodies, they may question their moral worth and agency, rather than simply lose bodily integrity. Women who miscarry can become distrustful of whether they ever had any moral responsibility for a fetus whose death is deemed insignificant by others.

As many feminists have argued, the dominant construction of pregnant bodies in modern obstetrics is that of a female body and a fetus who is a second patient (Mattingly 1992, 17; Rothman 1989, 160; Overall 1993, 40–41).[20] Women who receive obstetrical care learn to redescribe their bodily perspectives against that construction. North American women confront the image of the fetus as a separate entity during ultrasound examination, and not only because the technology gives them an actual image of the fetus, with them "nowhere in view" (Overall 1993, 41). In North America especially, physicians and sonographers often relate to the fetus of the ultrasound image as though it were an active, independent, and socialized agent (Mitchell and Georges 1998). For example, they describe fetal movement as "'playing,' 'swimming,' 'dancing,' 'partying,' and 'waving'" (108). They make comments about the fetus's personality, such as its shyness or cooperativeness (109).

The obstetrical construction of fetuses as separate from pregnant women can contradict women's own perspectives on their pregnant embodiment. Women experience such embodiment as the gradual differentiation between themselves and the fetus, according to Mackenzie. "From the perspective of the woman, the foetus becomes more and more physically differentiated from her as her own body boundaries alter" (Mackenzie 1992, 148–149). So in early stages of pregnancy, the fetus is more like a part of the woman than a distinct entity. Now that may not be true for all women, especially those with unwanted pregnancies, who may perceive their fetus initially as an alien being that has invaded their bodies. However, what is often alien for women in the early stages of wanted pregnancies is the idea that the fetus is somehow separate from them. Consequently, they can experience an early ultrasound performed in the way that Mitchell and Georges (1998) described as an assault on their bodily integrity.

With a sonographer's attention focused on the fetus as an independent and active agent, a woman can also feel (and be) objectified by an ultrasound examination. The more that the fetus is defined as separate from her, the more she becomes merely "the maternal environment." Such a self-perception is inconsistent with a decision to be morally responsible for her fetus as well as for herself. A passive environment cannot be morally responsible for anything; it is merely a backdrop against which others can be responsible for one another (i.e., against which a sonographer or physician can care for her and for the second patient). The effect of such objectification can be loss of bodily integrity as well as self-distrust about one's own moral role in pregnancy.

In the context of prenatal testing, some women face the image of themselves as hostile maternal environments, which can radically alter their perspective on their physical and moral relation to their fetus. Consider Carola's response to amniocentesis: "I cried for two days after I had the test. I guess I was identifying with universal motherhood; I felt like my image of my womb had been shattered. It still feels like it's in pieces, not like such a safe place as before. I guess technology gives us a certain kind of control, but we have to sacrifice something in return. I've lost my brash confidence that my body just produces healthy babies all by itself, naturally, and that if it doesn't, I can handle whatever comes along as a mother" (Rapp 1997, 131). Presumably, amniocentesis can be carried out in a way that is not as likely to cause such a harmful shift in a woman's bodily perspective. The test may be essentially destabilizing for women who perceive their bodies as places where healthy fetuses can grow; yet its destablizing effects are greatly enhanced when the person who performs it does not share that view. It seems that Carola's experience was mediated heavily by the perception that a woman's body is an unsafe place for a fetus, which the person testing her may have communicated by emphasizing the need for such tests and the problems they can uncover. Like women who are mere maternal environments, women who have bodies that are hostile toward fetuses cannot be morally responsible for them. They will inevitably cause them harm. Such a belief could ultimately explain why Carola lost her "brash confidence" in her ability to "handle whatever comes along as a mother." She might have reasoned that if she could not be responsible in pregnancy, how could she expect to be responsible in motherhood?

Thus, certain images of pregnancy and fetuses that pervade contexts involving prenatal testing can interfere with a woman's bodily integrity, a domain that overlaps with her moral integrity. One might ask why those images are so powerful for many women. The answer lies in the culturally sanctioned, epistemic authority of medicine. Such authority can lead to disintegrated bodily perspectives for women whose embodied knowledge of pregnancy, gained through their perception of what is happening in their bodies, conflicts with the supposedly disembodied knowledge of health care providers. In a contest over knowledge of the fetus between a woman and a health care provider, the woman usually loses, especially if the health care provider's claims are backed by medical technology. One woman told her sonographer, "We could see [the fetus] moving and . . . I felt it when I was taking the Metro. She said that wasn't it, that I couldn't feel it until a few more weeks. I thought for sure it was the baby moving, but I guess not" (Mitchell and Georges 1998, 110). A similar outcome in the contest over knowledge was described in chapter 3 between Janet, who claimed that she was pregnant, and her physician, who doubted her. By encouraging women to ignore or devalue their embodied knowledge of pregnancy, health care providers make it difficult for them to maintain coherent bodily perspectives. They continually have to explain away their own bodily experience, which can cause them to distrust their perception of their bodies and of what is happening in pregnancy.

Thus, the bodily integrity of pregnant women is endangered both by the conception of the fetus as a separate patient and by disrespect for a woman's embodied knowledge of pregnancy. The former can be a barrier as well to her self-respect and to trust in her own perception of where she stands morally in relation to her fetus. Both obstacles can encourage distrust in a woman's judgment about which beliefs concerning her pregnant embodiment should influence the choices she makes about her pregnancy.

Removing such obstacles would require fairly radical changes in obstetrical practice. It would require a shift toward what I call woman-centred obstetrics, in which fetuses are constructed in relation to pregnant women and some respect is given for women's embodied knowledge of pregnancy. Granted, in some obstetrical contexts it may be appropriate to view fetuses as separate (e.g., in fetal surgery); however, overall, they should not be defined as separate or independent entities. During ultrasound scanning, sonographers and physicians should try to avoid descriptions which suggest that they are self-sustaining beings.

Such a construction is morally problematic precisely because it can objectify pregnant women. However, it can be equally problematic to assume that all women in wanted pregnancies interpret their embodied relation to their fetus in the same way. We need a model of pregnancy as a relation, but not one that is so exact that it cannot accommodate varying degrees to which women view their fetuses as parts of them. Health care providers have to respect how individual women experience their pregnancies, rather than dictate to them what their experience is about. Whereas one might object that part of the job of an obstetrician is to offer women advice on how to perceive their pregnancies, surely they can do that without enforcing alienating bodily perspectives. And although they may have to negotiate with some patients about which perspectives to adopt, avoiding negotiation altogether and being authoritarian instead undermines patient self-trust and autonomy.

Similarly, in the contexts of miscarriage and abortion, it is important that health care providers be sensitive to the many ways that women might interpret pregnancies they lost or that they purposefully ended. However sympathetic health care providers are, they can cause harm by assuming that these women view their pregnancies in certain ways. Such assumptions can promote distrust in women's own perceptions of miscarriages or abortions, and that can interfere with autonomous behavior in overcoming those experiences or in truly understanding their personal significance.

When it comes to improving respect for women's embodied knowledge in pregnancy, substantial changes are necessary in medical epistemology. There is little room in that epistemology for embodied subjectivity (Foucault 1975); there is room only for "pure facts," known through objective scientific analysis and untainted by subjective views of physicians and researchers. Such an epistemology is not only implausible, it can lead to patients' loss of bodily integrity. Health care providers have to be aware that if they are dismissive of the embodied knowledge of pregnant women, they can compromise patients' bodily integrity as well as their autonomy. Instead, they should try to incorporate that knowledge as much as possible into the bodily perspectives they encourage pregnant women to adopt.

Where a Patient Trusts Herself too Much: The Role of Integrity-Preserving Persuasion

What if a pregnant woman trusts her embodied knowledge too much? Or, alternatively, what if she trusts herself to choose in ways that are divorced from an adequate conception of her own worth? In the former case, the woman might assume she is being responsible in trusting her perspective on what is happening in her body when in fact her perspective is unreliable. In this section I introduce the notion of "integrity-preserving" persuasion, or compromise (Benjamin 1990), as a way for physicians to deal with too much patient self-trust without destroying self-trust altogether. Preserving integrity helps to preserve self-trust, which is an attitude about one's own moral integrity.

First, I want to emphasize that health care providers are often not in a position to assess whether a patient has too much self-trust because she has an unrealistic conception of her own competencies or of her ability to cope with the consequences of a decision. Health care providers are not in that position in many obstetrical situations, including those involving prenatal testing and termination or continuation of a pregnancy. For example, if a woman decides to continue a pregnancy knowing that her child will have a genetic disorder and she has received ample information about raising such a child, normally only she and people close to her can judge whether her trust in that decision is justified.

Nonetheless, in some circumstances health care providers can evaluate whether a patient trusts herself too much because of inadequate self-knowledge. For example, if a woman decides to reduce her smoking dramatically during pregnancy without accepting any form of treatment, and she has often said in the past that she would quit but has never succeeded, her physician could probably conclude that her trust in that decision is unjustified. (Of course, that assumes that the woman has not been claiming to quit all along only to please or appease her physician.)

When it is clear that a patient trusts herself too much and in a way that could jeopardize her health or that of her fetus, health care providers could attempt persuasion that preserves integrity. This involves encouraging the patient to consider all of her values and beliefs, and how her current position may not reflect all of them accurately (Benjamin 1990). The aim "is to strengthen or encourage the recognition of [an] unacknowledged voice in the [patient]," rather than coerce her to take a position that is somehow alien (Benjamin 1990, 34). With the patient who trusts herself too much to quit smoking, the physician could assume that she knows she was unsuccessful in quitting in the past, and could ask her to reflect on that knowledge carefully. The physician could also assume that the patient values her own health and the health of her fetus, and that she knows that heavy smoking is hazardous to both of them. In other words, the physician could urge that from the patient's own perspective, it is important to choose a method of quitting that has the best chance of success. Such a strategy preserves integrity because the physician is trying to persuade the patient to adopt a position that is coherent, presumably, with the patient's own beliefs and values.

But, of course, the physician could be mistaken that the patient has certain latent desires or values that are unacknowledged in the decision she trusts so much. Say that a patient makes a choice that puts her own health at risk, but she is suffering from depression or has low self-worth. The physician might be wrong in assuming that she cares about her own health. Consider as well a patient who trusts her embodied perspective too much (e.g., she is adamant that she is not pregnant even though there is sufficient medical evidence to prove that she is). The physician might suspect, wrongly, that she values being responsible epistemically or that she believes that medical information and technology has some epistemic worth. Especially when the values and beliefs of patients and providers diverge dramatically (e.g., on whether medical technology has any epistemic value), it is unlikely that integrity-preserving persuasion will work.

Still an attempt at such persuasion is worth while particularly before recommending that a patient lose her decisional authority. Even with patients who trust themselves in ways that are incompatible with respect for their worth, integrity-preserving persuasion could have a positive effect. Since the voices of physicians are so powerful for some patients, it could be persuasive for a patient to hear from a physician that she deserves to be cared for well by herself and by others.

Where oppression or abuse has caused severe damage to a patient's self-worth or self-respect, however, it is doubtful that a physician alone could make inroads. In such cases, if the patient trusts a decision that puts her at grave risk of harm, counseling is appropriate, preferably with someone who is trained to help people with histories of psychological oppression or abuse.

Conclusion

Self-trust of a justified sort cannot be taken for granted among patients generally, not only among those who have been severely oppressed or abused. The attitude is essential if patients are to be autonomous. And while that is not the only requirement for patient autonomy, it is normally overlooked in philosophical and bioethical accounts of autonomy and informed choice. The value of self-trust has theoretical implications for the way that we conceive of autonomy. It also has profound practical implications for understanding the duty to respect patient autonomy, particularly in obstetrics. It is essential in obstetrics and other areas of reproductive medicine to acknowledge the importance of patient self-trust because of the enormous weight that oppression can bear on a woman's ability to trust herself in such contexts.

My suggestions for improving respect for patient autonomy in obstetrics go beyond what existing models of informed choice recommend, including the process model. Implicit in that model is the idea that patients should have sufficient time and information to assess their options; however, many barriers are more serious than lack of time or information. Many of them concern power imbalances in obstetrician-patient relationships that exist often because of the threat of oppressive stereotypes, or because of the authoritative epistemic position of obstetricians. The barrier of the construction of pregnancy as a relation between separate and distinct entities can interfere with patient self-trust at the level of determining one's authentic beliefs and values concerning one's relationship to one's fetus. Obstetricians and other health care providers should try to eliminate or at least minimize those barriers.

On the theoretical side of the relation between autonomy and self-trust, I have urged that while being able to trust oneself well is important for autonomy, so is being able to distrust oneself well. Self-distrust can avert the damage that hasty choices can have on our autonomy. Lara's case is an example of when self-distrust is justified, at least temporarily, with respect to a particular decision. Like most people, she is probably unreliable in trusting herself when forced to decide quickly about issues as complex as prenatal diagnosis. Still, if her self-distrust were to persist, it could threaten her autonomy. Too much self-distrust, even of a justified sort, is a barrier to autonomy.

Melissa's case is an example of where self-distrust is probably justified yet interferes with autonomy nonetheless. She does not trust herself to convince her obstetrician of her ability to make wise decisions about prenatal care because of the threat of being stereotyped negatively. Since members of stereotyped groups can animate stereotypes about them even while they strive to disconfirm their truth, it can be unreliable for them to trust themselves to succeed at that task. Stereotypes are more likely to be threatening if they are demeaning to those whom they target, and the most common targets of negative social stereotypes are oppressed people. Hence, there may be many more situations, in which it is unreliable for people who are oppressed to be self-trusting, whereas it is reliable for the privileged because of the influence of those stereotypes. As I observed in chapter 5, one's sociopolitical status tends to determine, in part, when it is reliable to trust or distrust.

Oppression as well as abuse can interfere with either the manifestation or the development of the ability to trust oneself well. Various mechanisms of oppression, such as stereotyping and objectifying, can encourage too much self-distrust in people who normally trust or distrust themselves well. Such mechanisms, together with abuse that is not oppression related, can prevent one from ever becoming a good self-truster or self-distruster. Some people who experienced childhood abuse or who live in an environment of severe oppression have never known what it is like to be self-trusting. Self-distrust is a constant feature of their lives and a constant impediment to settled opinions about what they truly believe and desire.

For that reason, if for no other, we have to acknowledge that self-trust and self-distrust are meaningful concepts and that we have a moral obligation to preserve and foster self-trust in one another. With those conceptual tools, we can then critically analyze the situation of patients, such as Lee, who are treated in reproductive health care contexts in ways that preclude or inhibit self-trust and consequently interfere with their reproductive autonomy—that is, with their ability to make authentic life choices about how and whether they will reproduce.

Reproductive autonomy, so defined, is something that many women still do not enjoy in Western society, and those who do may enjoy it even less than they did in the past because of new reproductive technologies. Much work remains to be done to ensure that women can be autonomous in reproductive health care. Disrespect for their perspectives on their pregnant bodies and for them as knowing subjects can promote such self-distrust that they lose control over what happens in pregnancy. With the relational account of self-trust, self-distrust, and autonomy I developed, we can make sense of why reproductive health care providers have a duty to allow women to trust themselves in the way most of them deserve to be trusted as autonomous agents.

Notes

Chapter 1

1. I use the pseudonym Lee to protect the privacy of this woman, with whom I am in personal contact and with whom I wrote an article on patient objectification in some fertility clinics (McLeod and Harris). Lee and I met at a time when she was searching for information as a way of understanding her experience, and I was researching this book. She shared her ordeal with me, together with her letters to her physicians, and for that I am truly honored and grateful. The quotations I give are from those letters.

2. That is a procedure done to determine if the fallopian tubes are blocked.

Chapter 2

1. I only assume that the "we" there are those of us in Western culture, and that the way "we" understand trust reflects the dominant uses of that term in "our" culture. Whereas subcultures in Western societies may interpret trust differently, and the way that "we" interpret it may overlap significantly with how it is understood in other cultures, I do not explore those possibilities here.

2. For example, in bioethics, see Edmund Pellegrino (1991) and Nancy Kass et al. (1996).

3. Prototype theory is not uncontroversial (see, e.g., Fodor 1998). I use it for two reasons: to exemplify a theory that allows more malleability to our concepts than the classical model; and to tie in my conceptual analysis of trust with a theory I develop in chapter 5, that trust is an emotion learned through association with paradigm scenarios, which are highly similar to prototypes. It makes sense that trust has a prototype structure if we learn when to trust or distrust in light of paradigm scenarios.

4. Hence, I speak later of the dominant trust prototype in our culture.

5. Still, for some people it may feel more natural to trust a dog than to trust human; an example is a child who has been neglected or physically abused.

6. By the second term, I do not mean that the relations are the prototypes rather than actual exemplars. They are prototypical in the sense that they inform our trust prototype.

7. Homosexual relationships are probably excluded because of the common oppressive stereotype that homosexuals are promiscuous. How could they possibly trust one another if that is the case (or so says the dominant view)?

8. This section is a version of my paper "Our Attitude Towards the Motivation of Those We Trust" (2000).

9. Disagreement comes from Richard Holton (1994), and ambiguity lies in Trudy Govier's *Dilemmas of Trust* (1998). She writes that when we trust someone, "we believe in his or her basic integrity; we are willing to rely on him or her," (91) and that when we trust ourselves, we have a firm belief in our "own good character and good sense" (95), or at least a "positive sense of our own motivation" (99). So do we want the trusted one to act with integrity, with good sense, with any kind of positive motivation, or with any motivation compatible with relying on someone?

10. Still, as I explain later, people we trust can be motivated entirely by kindly feelings as long as those feelings cohere with a commitment to do what is right.

11. Marcia Baron (1995) borrowed the primary-secondary motive distinction from Herman and concluded that the Kantian good will is structured in such a way that the agent's sense of duty plays a regulative function, as her secondary motive (129). In borrowing that distinction myself from Kantian theorists (i.e., Baron and Herman), I do not intend to suggest that the "commitment to act morally" that regulates the actions of persons with moral integrity is necessarily equivalent to a Kantian sense of duty. The commitment could just as easily entail an Aristotelian sense of virtue or a utilitarian's sense of moral obligation.

12. What it means to have an integrated self on those theories differs. Calhoun (1995, 236–252) explains in detail where the differences lie.

13. It is backward-looking in the sense that we assume responsibility for our causal role in creating a certain state of affairs. See Card (1996, 25–29) for a more detailed account of the distinction between forward and backward-looking responsibilities.

14. I do not pretend that it is typical for a woman to allow a physician to make decisions for her because she admires what the physician stands for. Substantial numbers of women in prenatal care may agree to what their physicians recommend because it seems easier to agree than to disagree. In other words, agreeing is the path of least resistance.

15. To quote Baier (1995, 123), when one relies on someone's "dependable habits, or only on their dependably exhibited fear, anger, or other motives compatible with ill will toward one," one is not trusting, but merely relying. But whether "dependable habits" can distinguish trust from mere reliance is questionable, as Diana Meyers pointed out to me in personal conversation. Moral integrity itself is probably a dependable habit since integrity is a virtue, and we tend

to form virtues out of habit. To use the language I do here, it is probably out of habit that people with moral integrity allow their commitment to doing what is right to regulate their primary motives for acting.

16. Cases where social sanctions allow for *mere* reliance are probably rare; usually, sanctions are not so restrictive that they require people to do exactly what we want them to do. Where gaps exist between our needs and what sanctions dictate, we have to trust that people will attend to our needs carefully.

17. Baier (1995) also thinks that trust can be morally rotten if the "truster relies on his threat advantage to keep the trust relation going." However, as I contend, if we manipulate others into doing what we rely on them to do, then we merely rely on them, not trust them.

18. She also added it as a feature of trusting attitudes to solve another problem: that we can rely on people to be benevolent and competent without trusting them. We only trust them, according to Jones (1996), once we expect them to be moved by the thought that we are counting on them. I disagree.

Chapter 3

1. Prototype theory states that we understand concepts in terms of prototypes of the phenomena to which our concepts refer, not in terms of necessary and sufficient conditions. For example, when we see some type of bird, we conceive of it as a bird because of its similarity to our prototype for bird (which is informed by different bird exemplars, such as robins or bluejays). We do not see a bird because the creature before us satisfies a set of necessary and sufficient conditions for being a bird.

2. That depends on what kind of test is performed and when it is performed. Blood tests are more sensitive in detecting the pregnancy hormone than urine tests, and modern urine tests will not detect the hormone at all before four weeks' gestation. Also, if a woman has what is called a missed abortion, in which the pregnancy has ended but there was no immediate miscarriage, the pregnancy test may be negative even though an ultrasound would show some trophoblastic tissue. (Source: Dr. Bruce Dunphy, reproductive endocrinologist, IWK-Grace Health Centre.)

3. Anne Fausto-Sterling (1985) made a similar claim in her work on scientific theories about sex differences. She pointed to the political motivations of scientists who are members of dominant groups to explain why they ignore perfectly good evidence in testing such hypotheses as, "women have poorer spatio-temporal abilities than men." It is clear that their political agendas shape what they deem to be actual evidence.

4. I return to that issue in chapter 7.

5. I claimed in chapter 2 that we can acknowledge that our own moral values are not entirely objective, which is how we can grant moral integrity to people whose moral values are somewhat different than ours. Expecting that of our

moral values is not the same as expecting that they will change in the near future. We can admit some uncertainty about the objectivity of our values, yet remain committed to them (if partly out of faith or habit, rather than reason).

6. Our society does not assume that it is second nature for all women. Oppressive stereotypes or negative presuppositions about some women's mothering abilities (including black women and those with disabilities) exclude them from that category.

7. There, I interpret "expectation" differently from even enormous optimism by assuming that the latter entails some awareness (conscious or unconscious) of the possibility of disappointment, whereas the former does not.

8. One might discern the relevant risks unconsciously. Caroline Whitbeck (1995, 2502) assumed otherwise and found that Luhmann's distinction between trust and confidence does not make room for unconscious trust. That is false if the knowledge of risks can be unconscious.

9. That is a conservative estimate from *Unsung Lullabies* (Leaney and Silver 1995). According to Rajan and Oakley (1993, 75), approximately 80% of pregnancies end in miscarriage. Note, however, that the number of miscarriages that women detect and therefore experience has undoubtedly increased over the years as the sensitivity and accuracy of pregnancy tests have increased.

10. One reason cited in the literature is inhibitions people in our culture have about discussing death (Rajan and Oakley 1993, 75, 81). People may even be less comfortable in acknowledging the death of a fetus than they are the death of a child or adult, because Western culture has no socially sanctioned rituals (e.g., attending a funeral service or sending flowers to the woman and her partner) for honoring the importance that a fetus (or potential future child) had in their lives.

11. Calling it a syndrome is not entirely appropriate, as the name suggests that something is wrong with the women rather than with a society that pressures women to take on so much responsibility.

12. According to Darwall (1995), not just any competency is a proper object of self-respect; the relevant competencies must reflect our moral character. It is not clear that all of the competencies we can trust ourselves to have would fit that description. For example, if I trust myself as a tree planter to be competent and committed to planting trees properly, my competency may not stem from my moral character. I may be competent only because I am physically capable of planting well.

13. Diana Meyers posed that objection to me in personal conversation.

14. People who have appraisal self-respect (i.e., optimism about their moral character) are more likely to be self-trusting than those who do not. And people who trust themselves are likely to build appraisal self-respect, as they give themselves the chance to prove their character and competency to themselves.

15. Here, I draw on my own experience of having a miscarriage in an unwanted pregnancy (an experience that is underrepresented in the literature on miscarriage). I also appeal to a study showing that the levels of depression for women

who have miscarried in unwanted pregnancies can equal those for women who lose wanted pregnancies (Neugebauer et al. 1992).

16. See Dorothy Roberts (1997, 15): "American culture upholds no popular image of a black mother tenderly nurturing her child."

17. In fact, Anna's partner may have been truly sympathetic without knowing quite how to express that. It is common for men to be confused about how they should behave toward their partners who miscarry (Puddifoot and Johnson 1997).

18. As Campbell (1997, 108) explained, "uptake in collaborative individuation [can be] facilitated by . . . overlapping biographies [or] personal knowledge." Thus, the best listeners for women who miscarry are often people who themselves have miscarried or who have intimate knowledge of how women can respond emotionally to this event.

A study by Lynda Rajan and Ann Oakley (1993) showed an appreciable difference in the emotional health of women who received good emotional support after miscarriage compared with those who did not. They recommended that women be offered support from someone who is trained to respond well to their emotional needs. However, it is also important that primary health care providers receive training for this, as they could cause harm by responding in insensitive ways.

Chapter 4

1. However, trust is relevant beyond situations of vulnerability, as I imply in this chapter. For example, some instances in which a parent cultivates trust in a child may be related solely to the child's moral education rather than to the parent's vulnerability.

2. Trust is also relevant beyond situations where we incur vulnerability, such as when we trust without expecting the trusting one to show specific concern for us. See chapter 2, where I distinguish between trust with specific concern and trust without specific concern.

3. In chapter 7 I discuss what bodily integrity means, specifically in the context of pregnancy.

4. It is also difficult in theory when trust is unwelcome. When someone does not welcome my trust and does not act in accordance with it, does she betray me or merely disappoint me? That would depend it seems on the accuracy of her perception of the nature of our relationship. As I stated, trust is unwelcome when the trusted one does not perceive her relationship with me as the kind that requires her to fulfill the responsibility I trust her to fulfill. But she could be wrong about the nature of our relationship. By encouraging me to have certain expectations and by behaving in certain ways toward me, she may have unwittingly established a relationship that she thought she avoided. In that case, if she does not satisfy my trust, she betrays it, even though it was unwanted.

5. That is not necessarily true in the former case; if it turns out that the trusted person does not hold the relevant values, it cannot violate her integrity for her to fail to act on those values.

6. See, especially, Johnston (1998) and Rorty (1994, 1998).

7. Such embodiment occurs with people who are abused when they think of themselves as mere bodies as a way of enduring the violation to their selves.

8. I develop the point that caring for women who abuse drugs in pregnancy is morally preferable to incarcerating them in "Women's Autonomy and the 'G' Case" (1998).

9. That point comes ultimately from Walker (1998, 76, 77): "social privileges of others permit (and perhaps contain or deflect the effects of) irresponsible, craven, or dishonorable commitments and actions."

10. On the mistaken idea that black people abuse drugs more often than whites, see Eva Marie Smith (1993). On the mistaken view that black women make bad mothers, Dorothy Roberts (1997) outlined various disparaging myths and described how they are perpetuated in the media and elsewhere (see, especially, Introduction).

11. One could say that rather than being deceived by the condition of being emotionally well-adjusted, people who have that condition are cultivating self-trust in a way that prompts (self-)trustworthiness (Diana Meyers, personal communication). However, I assume that it is a contested matter whether people with positive outlooks are able to honor their trust as frequently (or nearly as frequently) as they bestow it on themselves. Some might appear to have that ability even though their privilege is buoying them up, making them only seem trustworthy to themselves. Privilege can allow people to "duck or hand off to others" difficult or conflicting responsibilities (Walker 1998, 78); and sometimes, people do not realize how much ducking they are doing, or how much their capacity to meet their commitments stems directly from their privilege.

12. Yet the prototypes can be good guides if an oppressive upbringing denied one the opportunity to develop the competence and integrity necessary for justified self-trust in some domains. I discuss that idea in chapter 5.

Chapter 5

1. That epistemology focuses on when *persons* are justified in trusting themselves or others, not about whether trust is justified in some abstract sense. Modern epistemology notes a distinction between what John Pollock (1979) called subjective and objective justification. Subjective justification is meant to capture the intuition that someone could be justified in believing X even though the means used to arrive at X are faulty (an example is the appeal to oracles and astrology in predicting the future; Goldman 1992, 127, 128). If those means are culturally sanctioned, we would want to be able to say that the belief is justified *for that person,* even though we would not say that it is justified overall (i.e., objectively speaking). But is it really meaningful to say that something is justified overall, ir-

respective of any person? Many epistemologists, in particular feminists, reject the "view from nowhere" as a potential source of justification (Nagel 1986). Justification always comes from somewhere and is always for someone, and it is not necessarily subjective as a result, in the sense of lacking objectivity. In arguing that trusting attitudes are justified relative to someone's sociopolitical position, I am not speaking of subjective justification; that is, something less pure than objective justification.

2. A possible exception is when trust is cultivated. Cultivating trust, which I describe later, may be purely strategic.

3. The fact that emotions are more "informationally encapsulated" than beliefs, as I explain, implies that we can be justified in having emotions in the face of contrary evidence, at least until we have time to process that evidence. The processing time must be longer with emotions than with beliefs, given the greater resistance of emotions to contrary evidence.

4. It is not to say that emotions have only those elements. A complete account of emotions would explain what apart from their perceptual and behavioral dimensions gives them the identity of emotions, an example being some physiological change or "disturbance" in the agent (to use a term of Paul Griffiths 1997).

5. Only attitudes involving some appraisal of our situation are subject to rational evaluation. The relevant attitudes can be representational not by chance, in other words, but only through use of our evaluative capacities.

6. It seems that for de Sousa (1987), cognitive does mean simply representational: "the term [cognition] must be taken to imply the existence of some objective correlation between some representational state and some object in the real world" (41). He aimed to show that "emotions carry information about the world beyond the subject, although . . . they are not species of beliefs" (41). Hence, they are cognitive (in his sense), but they do not necessarily have propositional objects. Rorty (1980, 112) similarly rejected tradition and made room for a species of cognitive attitudes that are nonpropositional.

7. Further elaboration on the nature of these sets would lend further support to my thesis in favor of a reliabilist theory of the justification of trust and distrust. The cognitive sets that underlie emotions tend to be "submersed; . . . emotional 'seeings of the world as' resist alteration largely because we lack a clear view of the cognitive set operative in these 'seeings as . . . '" (Calhoun 1984, 341). And even if we had a clear view, it would be difficult consciously to evaluate such cognitive frameworks because of how complex they tend to be. Thus, it would seem that epistemic internalism about emotional attitudes is implausible. I make that claim about an internalist theory of the justification of trust and distrust. The complex factors that go into our trusting and distrusting attitudes are beyond our reflective access and beyond reflective evaluation.

8. We can identify clear methods for cultivating trust, but not for developing justified attitudes of trust and distrust, as I discuss. I suspect that the way that cultivating trust is justified is complicated. I reserve discussion of that issue for another time.

9. The woman's bootstrapping would not make her oblivious to relevant counter-evidence. Accepting that her attitude is a belief would involve accepting that beliefs can be formed in the face of what the subject acknowledges to be substantial counter-evidence. But the preponderance of discussion in the literature on beliefs opposes that view; we cannot have beliefs without regard for what we perceive to be evidence for or against them.

10. It is important that I never assumed the need to trust Jan because it is possible that I have a dispositional attitude of trust toward her. I might trust her, but not currently. We can probably rule that out, however, if my life and hers are entirely separate.

11. Surely, we distinguish between acting with moral character and acting because we are forced or coerced. Such a distinction collapses for some social contract theorists who are psychological egoists and therefore believe that we never could act morally in the absence of external reward or punishment. However, psychological egoism is a profoundly problematic doctrine (Feinberg 1978).

12. One might say that Baier is right that rationality has to do with rule following, and hence, that I am confusing rationality with justification. One might say that whereas it is sensible to talk about justification being independent of rules for forming attitudes about the world, that is not true for rationality. The latter always has a strategic element to it, whether or not its teleology is epistemic, and that element demands that we provide set rules for decision making. Although many rational decision theorists might agree with that view, it is too narrow. We sometimes do think of rationality merely as a success term: an attitude is rational if it is likely to target its intentional object successfully (see de Sousa 1987, 159). Moreover, "we typically scrutinize [origins] in order to access whether a state or action is *likely* to [be successful]" (de Sousa 1987, 161–162). Thus, a view of epistemic rationality that looks to origins and to whether an attitude or state represents the world right is comprehensible. Epistemic rationality can be modeled on an externalist epistemology.

13. Mark Johnston held that self-deception does not even occur on an intentional level; rather, it occurs on what he called a "sub-intentional level" (1988).

14. See also William Ruddick (1988) and Rom Harre (1988).

15. Feedback can come from a variety of sources especially in democratic countries where art and the media are not as censored as they are elsewhere. With access to politically progressive films and literature, for example, we can dilute whatever poisoning influence oppressive norms and stereotypes have on attitudes of trust and distrust.

16. Nonetheless, the degree to which we are justified in trusting cannot equal the degree to which we are justified in distrusting; in that case, the only attitude we are justified in adopting is one of neutrality.

17. There, most of the feedback would be indirect; it would be what she received about her past self-trusting attitudes. Generally, we decide whether to be distrusting depending on how successful we were in the past in trusting. And often we know of that success (or the lack of it) because often when our trusting atti-

tudes are mistaken they run smack against the world. That is, we experience harm or disappointment immediately in ways that make it obvious to us that we have gotten things wrong. We seldom discover, by contrast, whether our distrust is mistaken, for whatever harms it makes us vulnerable to tend not to be immediate (e.g., the harm of foregoing valuable relationships with people of certain social groups because of distrust that is laced with bigotry).

18. Psychological studies attempting to prove that disparity provide evidence that the stereotype exists. A well-known example is the Kohlberg study, which Carol Gilligan criticized (1987).

19. A standard objection to reliabilism is that it is impossible to define reliability and the "normal" conditions to which it is indexed in a nonarbitrary way (Pollock 1986, 118–120). For example, where I said that Eve's self-distrust is justified, it seems equally plausible to say that the processes responsible for it are unreliable. It is tempting to claim that although normally they are reliable, they are unreliable in circumstances involving deception. However, it is equally tempting to assert that even in such circumstances they are reliable because normally they produce attitudes that are well grounded. So how can we decide, nonarbitrarily, which description of those processes to accept? Answering that objection demands a lot of epistemological work (focused specifically on reliabilism, not trust). I demonstrate here that an adequate answer must attend to the various ways in which reliability is relativized to the subject's social position.

However, given the severity of the objection, let me say something brief in response. I do not think that, for most of us, it is as tempting to say that the conditions Eve faces in the last scenario I described are normal, compared with conditions in which no one hoodwinks her. Normal conditions tell us whether the agent should have been able to trust herself or trust others well, something that we tend to understand in light of social (and sometimes, moral) norms. The norm that deception is prima facie wrong, for example, informs our sense that Eve should have been able to trust herself; the forces that prevented it made her self-distrust justified. If social norms play a role in defining reliability, knowledge will be somewhat localized to a system of norms. However, it need not be entirely local, for we do have the means to criticize such norms, means that within some feminist epistemologies involve engaging with people at the margins of society, who are likely to have a more objective perspective on dominant social norms than we do.

20. We would have to make the distinction without buying into the objective/subjective split of mainstream epistemology discussed in note 1 of this chapter.

Chapter 6

1. The degree to which people must do that can vary. I explain later that autonomy can admit of degrees and that the degree to which one has to trust oneself reliably to be autonomous depends on what level of autonomy we have in mind.

2. See Seyla Benhabib (1987), Carol Pateman (1988), Lorraine Code (1991), and Alison Jaggar (1983). For complete lists of different feminist critiques of autonomy, see Catriona Mackenzie and Natalie Stoljar (2000, Introduction) and

Marilyn Friedman (1997). Diana Meyers (1989, part II, section I) discussed the presocial self that underlies many contemporary theories of autonomy (including the views in moral philosophy that I discuss later). Those theories presuppose that kind of self, as Meyers explained, because they interpret autonomy as a kind of free will that demands transcendence above the level of socialization.

3. The phrase "pathological or infantile" comes from Susan Dodds (2000, 214). She and Anne Donchin (1995) criticized the standard conception of autonomy in bioethics for being individualistic in the sense that I describe immediately after this note (Donchin 2000, 237).

4. Examples of the moral philosophers are Dworkin (1989, 61) and Young (1989, 81). Young focused specifically on ignorance that stems from self-deception. Although philosophers such as him acknowledge ignorance as a potential obstacle to autonomy, they (unlike the bioethicists) do not say explicitly that understanding the nature of one's options is an important condition for autonomy.

5. Having that much order in our lives would surely be a detriment as far as our autonomy goes. We would be obsessed with perfecting our plans and lose valuable time for actualizing them. I support Meyers's (1989, 49–53) view of how planned out an autonomous life must be.

6. And this does not necessarily presuppose either a transparent or a unified self, as some feminist philosophers presume. Knowing one's self—one's values, beliefs, identity—is a social process, as I stated in chapter 4, precisely because the self is not transparent through introspection.

7. There are a number of reasons why lesbians are often denied that option, the most obvious of which is that fertility clinics will refuse them access (Murphy 1999, 105, citing Robinson 1997).

8. With ovarian hyperstimulation, the woman takes hormone injections to stimulate her ovaries to produce several eggs in one cycle, rather than the usual one egg. The rationale is that the more eggs and sperm that interact, the greater the chances of conception (source: patient information leaflet).

9. There may even be further options of using donor sperm and donor eggs, and of having preimplantation genetic diagnosis, which is "no longer a futuristic technique" (Donchin 2000, 250). That procedure is designed to minimize the chance of having a child with certain genetic abnormalities.

10. Some of those drugs are estrogen based, and correlation between estrogen and breast cancer is well known. Furthermore, women who have twelve or more cycles of drug-induced ovulation have an elevated risk of developing ovarian tumors (Rossing et al. 1994).

Fillion also noted the possible risk of childhood cancer. "A review of Japan Children's Cancer Register from 1985–89 identified significantly more cases of childhood malignant disease in children born to mothers who underwent ovulation induction" (1994, 55, ftn 2).

11. See the *Globe & Mail* (May 24, 1999, A1, A6, A7; May 22, 1999, A1, A8, A9). In response to the outrage, the federal government in Canada proposed new legislation requiring IVF clinics to release live birth rates.

12. Being cancelled means that you miss a cycle, not that you are kicked out of the program altogether. However, missing a cycle can be devastating enough either because a woman may have placed all of her hopes in conceiving in one particular cycle, or she may not have the financial means to try again (patients have to pay separately for each cycle).

13. A number of writers described in some detail how stressful IVF can be (Shanner 1996; Fillion 1994; Williams 1989). For a detailed account of what the procedure involves medically, see Farquhar (1996, chapter 5).

14. The clinic I attended as part of my clinical practicum provides no counseling service. The Canadian Royal Commission on New Reproductive Technologies recommended that counseling be made available at all clinics as a means of avoiding any "unexpected consequences" of the new technologies (1993, 4).

15. While Joanne's story is somewhat dated, it is consistent with more recent reports about what many women, and men, experience emotionally during IVF (Fillion 1994; Mentor 1998; Shanner 1996; *Globe & Mail* reports cited in note 11). One man said, "Every month for three days it's like a funeral. We've had twenty-four funerals. If she does get pregnant, I'm not going to feel that something is beginning. I'm going to feel 'Thank God it's over'" (Fillion 1994, 33).

16. Morgan (1989) acknowledged that not all women experience that dimension of sexism in every domain, and some (e.g., lesbians and poor women) are often pressured by the dominant culture in the opposite direction, that is, not to reproduce (see Roberts 1997). Still, within their own communities, lesbians and poor women can experience fertility as obligatory (Morgan 1989, 78).

17. That choice becomes even more complex once we factor in implications for the value of children already living who are homeless or are in foster care, and also for the value of children conceived using ARTs, who may be commodified in the process.

18. In a later paper, Meyers (2000, 176, ftn. 23) said that drawing a sharp line between moral and personal autonomy is impossible "because different domains of autonomous choice and action overlap." She holds on to the distinction nonetheless.

19. But if their talents were simply hidden, cultivating self-trust would probably improve their autonomy. For people who are actually incompetent, however, it is not clear that cultivated self-trust would further their autonomy.

Chapter 7

1. The closest approximation I have seen to such a recommendation is in the work of Abby Wilkerson (1998, 133): "Women need to be able to trust our own perceptions of our bodies and our experiences, a goal that medical theory and practice should respect and support."

2. That is what is supposed to happen with genetic testing for fetal abnormalities: patients are meant to be told that they have the option of having maternal

serum screening and, possibly, also amniocentesis or chorionic villus sampling (see the case of Lara). However, I have certainly encountered physicians who recommend testing rather than offer it, particularly for women who are at higher risk than average of having a fetus with a genetic abnormality.

3. In their study they did not find significant ethnic or class differences in women's attitudes toward the medical advice they received about pregnancy. However, they acknowledge that other anthropologists or sociologists have documented such differences (e.g., Kay 1980; Lazarus 1994; Rapp 1993).

4. Physicians are meant to do only preliminary assessments of decisional capacity and to recommend psychiatric consultation for a patient who seems to lack that capacity.

5. Such teams are particularly common in fertility clinics in Canada, although I have encountered them in clinics that deal with women's health concerns in general. In a paper that I wrote with Lee Harris (n.d.), we criticize the kind of team approach to which she was subjected because of how it objectifies patients.

6. Versions of the test vary depending on how many markers are analyzed. The triple screen is meant to be most effective; it tests the serum levels of three different substances. Still, its false positive rates are high (they are the rates I gave above; see Mennuti 1996, 1442–1443).

7. In my experience doing the clinical practicum, it was rare for men to be present at prenatal visits unless an ultrasound was scheduled or unless their partner was having a difficult procedure done, such as amniocentesis.

8. These are the options and the risks for a 37-year-old woman who is receiving prenatal care at the IWK Grace Health Centre in Halifax (Barbara Parish, personal communication, 1999). Michael Mennuti (1996) also cited the same risks that I give for diagnostic procedures.

9. Ann Donchin (2000, 250) writes, "for [women's] partners, prenatal diagnosis is often a less immediate worry, more easily postponed or denied."

10. That concern is common among woman in the hospital where I did my practicum, according to nurse Diane O'Reilly, who works in grief counseling for women who have had pregnancies terminated because of fetal abnormalities (personal communication, 1998).

11. In medical contexts where it is not obvious that patients have a moral responsibility to choose one option over another, on the other hand, health care providers should *not* support each option equally. Consider a woman who is HIV-positive and has the option of taking a drug during pregnancy that would significantly reduce the risk of viral transmission to the fetus. Her physician would be remiss in giving as much support to refusal as to consent (which should not be confused with the act of revoking the former option). But prenatal diagnosis is not a situation of that sort (i.e., one where it is clear where the woman's moral responsibilities lie) and neither is infertility treatment, for example.

12. One study showed that 75% of women feel that they would not be able to refuse an offer of prenatal diagnosis (Sjogren and Uddenberg 1988, cited in Gates

1994, 188). Sometimes, it is assumed that middle-class women accept testing more often than working-class women, which suggests that the former might feel more obligated than the latter to accept it (Rapp 1998, 148). However, if poor women have access to a clinic where they feel comfortable and trust their health care providers, they are just as likely as middle-class women to consent to prenatal diagnosis (Rapp 1998, 149, 150). Hence, the disparity in the rates of their refusal compared with middle-class women often has more to do with inadequate prenatal care services for poor women than with their attitudes toward testing.

13. That is true for all mosaic conditions, in which fetal cells are "both normal and atypical in varying proportions" (Rapp 1998, 163). It is also true that the disabling conditions of some genetic anomalies are completely unknown to geneticists (see Rapp 1998, 161, 162).

14. One could contend that many people with disabilities lead rewarding and productive lives, and that they enrich our society by offering perspectives on what is important in life that others lack. Those who find such notions unpersuasive and firmly believe that it is in society's interest to prevent disability should at least express that interest in a way that does not further stigmatize and oppress people currently living with disabilities. See Laurie Nsiah-Jefferson (1994, 234) on how the very availability of prenatal diagnosis can perpetuate ableism.

15. Some American authors, such as Alto Charo and Karen Rothenberg (1994, 111), pointed out that although pressure on women to have prenatal diagnosis is increasing in the United States, access to adequate abortion services and counseling is decreasing.

16. I am not thinking of cases in which subordinate groups reclaim terms, such as "fag" or "Indian," and define themselves proudly using them. I am thinking of cases in which people mock stereotypes: e.g., a woman who "acts like a lady" as a joke.

17. I learned of Steele's studies from Walker (1998, 196, 197). They focus primarily on black students in the United States, and show that while writing exams they can develop intense anxiety about whether their results will confirm the stereotype of blacks as less intelligent than whites. The anxiety inhibits them from performing well.

18. Obviously, health care professionals alone should not have that responsibility, especially in deflating stereotypes about oppressed people. However, they can play a role in reducing the negative effects of those stereotypes.

19. Many philosophers use the term "bodily integrity" in that way to defend a woman's right to refuse unwanted interventions in pregnancy, or simply to refuse to continue unwanted pregnancies (Mackenzie 1992; Warren 1975; Overall 1987).

20. Many textbooks on obstetrics confirm the patient status of fetuses in their titles: examples are *The Unborn Patient: Prenatal Diagnosis and Treatment* (Harrison et al. 1990) and *The Fetus as a Patient* (Kurjak 1985).

References

Alden, Paulette Bates. 2000. "From *Crossing the Moon*." In *Bearing Life: Women's Writings on Childlessness*. Ed. Rochelle Ratner. New York: Feminist Press.

Alderman, Loraine, June Chisholm, Florence Denmark, and Stephen Salbod. 1998. "Bereavement and Stress of a Miscarriage: As It Affects the Couple," *Omega: Journal of Death and Dying* 37(4): 317–327.

Appelbaum, Paul and Loren Roth. 1982. "Competency to Consent to Research: A Psychiatric Overview," *Archives of General Psychiatry* 39: 951–958.

Babbitt, Susan. 1996. *Impossible Dreams: Rationality, Integrity, and Moral Imagination*. Boulder: Westview.

Baier, Annette. 1985. *Postures of the Mind: Essays on Mind and Morals*. Minneapolis: University of Minnesota Press.

———. 1995. *Moral Prejudices: Essays on Ethics*. Cambridge: Harvard University Press.

Baker, Judith. 1987. "Trust and Rationality," *Pacific Philosophical Quarterly* 68: 1–13.

———. 1996. "Trusting Relations." Presented at the Canadian Philosophical Association annual conference (May).

Baron, Marcia. 1995. *Kantian Ethics Almost without Apology*. Ithaca: Cornell University Press.

Bartky, Sandra Lee. 1990. *Femininity and Domination: Studies in the Phenomenology of Oppression*. New York: Routledge.

Baylis, Francoise. 1993. "Assisted Reproductive Technologies: Informed Choice." In *New Reproductive Technologies: Ethical Aspects*. Vol. 1 of the research studies of the Royal Commission on New Reproductive Technologies. Ottawa: Minister of Supply and Services Canada.

———, Jocelyn Downie, and Susan Sherwin. 1998. "Reframing Research Involving Humans." In *The Feminist Health Care Ethics Research Network*. The politics of Woman's Health: Exploring Agency and Astronomy. Philadelphia: Temple University Press.

Beauchamp, Tom and James Childress. 1994. *Principles of Biomedical Ethics,* 4th ed. Oxford: Oxford University Press.

Benhabib, Seyla. 1987. "The Generalized and the Concrete Other: The Kohlberg-Gilligan Controversy and Feminist Theory." In *Feminism as Critique.* Eds. Seyla Benhabib and Drucilla Cornell. Minneapolis: University of Minnesota Press.

Benjamin, Martin. 1990. *Splitting the Difference: Compromise and Integrity in Ethics and Politics.* Lawrence: University Press of Kansas.

Benson, Paul. 1994. "Free Agency and Self-worth," *Journal of Philosophy* 91(12): 650–668.

Boetzkes, Elizabeth. 1999. "Equality, Autonomy, and Feminist Bioethics." In Donchin and Purdy, eds.

Brison, Susan. 1997. "Outliving Oneself: Trauma, Memory, and Personal Identity." In Meyers: 12–39.

Brothers, Doris. 1982. "Trust Disturbances in Rape and Incest-Victims." Ph.D. dissertation, Yeshiva University, New York.

Browner, Carole and Nancy Press. 1995. "The Normalization of Prenatal Diagnostic Testing." In *The Politics of Reproduction.* Eds. Faye Ginsburg and Rayna Rapp. Berkeley: University of California Press.

———. 1997. "The Production of Authoritative Knowledge in American Prenatal Care." In *Childbirth and Authoritative Knowledge: Cross-Cultural Perspectives.* Eds. Robbie Davis-Floyd and Carolyn Sargent. Berkeley: University of California Press.

Calhoun, Cheshire. 1984. "Cognitive Emotions?" In *What Is an Emotion?* Eds. Cheshire Calhoun and Robert C. Solomon. New York: Oxford University Press.

———. 1995. "Standing for Something," *Journal of Philosophy* 92(5): 235–260.

Campbell, Richmond. 1998. *Illusions of Paradox: A Feminist Epistemology Naturalized.* Lanham: Rowman & Littlefield.

Campbell, Sue. 1997. *Interpreting the Personal: Expression and the Formation of Feelings.* Ithaca: Cornell University Press.

Card, Claudia. 1996. *The Unnatural Lottery: Character and Moral Luck.* Philadelphia: Temple University Press.

Charo, R. Alta and Karen Rothenberg. 1994. " 'The Good Mother': The Limits of Reproductive Accountability and Genetic Choice." In Rothenberg and Thomson, eds.

Chasnoff, Ira J., Harvey J. Landress, and Mark E. Barrett. 1990. "The Prevalence of Illicit-Drug or Alcohol Use During Pregnancy and Discrepancies in Mandatory Reporting in Pinellas County, Florida," *New England Journal of Medicine* 322: 1202–1206.

Christman, John, ed. 1989. *The Inner Citadel: Essays on Individual Autonomy.* Oxford: Oxford University Press.

———. 1991. "Autonomy and Personal History," *Canadian Journal of Philosophy* 21: 1—24.

Churchland, Paul. 1996. "The Neural Representation of the Social World." In May et al., eds.

Clark, Andy. 1996. "Connectionism, Moral Cognition, and Collaborative Problem Solving." In May et al., eds.

Code, Lorraine. 1991. "Second Persons." In *What Can She Know? Feminist Theory and the Construction of Knowledge.* Ithaca: Cornell University Press.

Darwall, Stephen. 1995. "Two Kinds of Self-Respect." In *Dignity, Character, and Self-Respect.* Ed. Robin Dillon. New York: Routledge.

Davis-Floyd, Robbie. 1992. *Birth as an American Rite of Passage.* Berkeley: University of California Press.

Davis-Floyd, Robbie, and Joseph Dumit, eds. 1998. *Cyborg Babies: From Techno-Sex to Techno-Tots.* New York: Routledge.

Deigh, John. 1983. "Shame and Self-Esteem: A Critique," *Ethics* 93: 225–245.

de Sousa, Ronald. 1987. *The Rationality of Emotion.* Cambridge: MIT Press.

Dillon, Robin. 1992. "Toward A Feminist Conception of Self-Respect," *Hypatia* 7: 52–69.

———. 1997. "Self-Respect: Moral, Emotional, Political," *Ethics* 107: 226–249.

Dodds, Susan. 2000. "Choice and Control in Feminist Bioethics." In Mackenzie and Stoljar, eds.

Donchin, Anne. 1995. "Reworking Autonomy: Toward a Feminist Perspective," *Cambridge Quarterly of Healthcare Ethics* 4(1): 44–55.

———. 2000. "Autonomy and Interdependence: Quandries in Genetic Decision Making." In Mackenzie and Stoljar, eds.

Donchin, Anne and Laura Purdy, eds. 1999. *Embodying Bioethics: Recent Feminist Advances.* Lanham: Rowman & Littlefield.

Dworkin, Gerald. 1989. "Autonomy, Science, and Morality." In Christman, ed.

Faden, Ruth and Tom Beauchamp. 1986. *A History and Theory of Informed Consent.* Oxford: Oxford University Press.

Farquhar, Dion. 1996. *The Other Machine: Discourse and Reproductive Technologies.* New York: Routledge.

Fausto-Sterling, Anne. 1985. *Myths of Gender: Biological Theories about Women and Men.* New York: Basic Books.

Feinberg, Joel. 1978. "Psychological Egoism." In *Reason and Responsibility,* 4th ed. Belmont, CA: Wadsworth.

Fillion, Kate. 1994. "Fertility Rights, Fertility Wrongs." In *Misconceptions: The Social Construction of Choice and the New Reproductive and Genetic Technologies.* Eds. Gwynne Basen, Margrit Eichler, and Abby Lippman. Vol. 2. Hull, Quebec: Voyageur Publishing.

Flanagan, Owen. 1996. "Ethics Naturalized: Ethics as Human Ecology." In May et al., eds.

Fodor, Jerry. 1998. *Concepts: Where Cognitive Science Went Wrong*. Oxford: Clarendon Press.

Foucault, Michel. 1975. *The Birth of the Clinic*. Trans. A.M. Sheridan Smith. New York: Vintage Books.

Frankfurt, Harry. 1989. "Freedom of the Will and the Concept of a Person." In Christman, ed.

Friedman, Marilyn. 1986. "Autonomy and the Split-level Self," *Southern Journal of Philosophy* 24: 19–35.

———. 1997. "Autonomy and Social Relationships: Rethinking the Feminist Critique." In Meyers, ed.

Frye, Marilyn. 1983. "In and Out of Harm's Way: Arrogance and Love." In *The Politics of Reality: Essays in Feminist Theory*. Freedom: Crossing Press.

Gates, Elena. 1994. "Prenatal Genetic Testing: Does it Benefit Pregnant Women?" In Rothenberg and Thomson, eds.

Gilligan, Carol. 1987. In a Different Voice. Cambridge: Harvard University Press.

Goldman, Alvin. 1992. *Liaisons: Philosophy Meets the Cognitive and Social Sciences*. Cambridge, MA: MIT Press.

———. 1999. "Internalism Exposed," *Journal of Philosophy* 96(6): 271–293.

Govier, Trudy. 1993a. "An Epistemology of Trust," *International Journal of Moral and Social Studies* 8(2): 155–174.

———. 1993b. "Self-Trust, Autonomy, and Self-Esteem," *Hypatia* 8(1): 99–120.

———. 1998. *Dilemmas of Trust*. Montreal and Kingston: McGill-Queen's University Press.

Griffiths, Paul. 1997. *What Emotions Really Are: The Problem of Psychological Categories*. Chicago: University of Chicago Press.

Hardin, Russell. 1996. "Trustworthiness," *Ethics* 107: 26–42.

Harre, Rom. 1988. "The Social Context of Self-Deception." In McLaughlin and Rorty. eds.

Harrison, Michael R., Mitchell S. Golbus, and Roy A. Filly, eds. 1990. *The Unborn Patient: Prenatal Diagnosis and Treatment*, 2nd ed. Philadelphia: Saunders.

Herman, Barbara. 1981. "On the Value of Acting from the Motive of Duty," *Philosophical Review* 90:359–382.

Herman, Judith Lewis. 1992. *Trauma and Recovery*. New York: Basic Books.

Hey, Valerie, Catharine Itzin, Lesley Saunders, and Mary Anna Speakman. 1996. *Hidden Loss: Miscarriage and Ectopic Pregnancy*, 2nd ed. London, UK: Women's Press.

Holton, Richard. 1994. "Deciding to Trust, Coming to Believe," *Australasian Journal of Philosophy* 72:63–76.

Jaggar, Alison. 1983. *Feminist Politics and Human Nature*. Brighton: Harvester Press.

James, D.S. and C.M. Kristiansen. 1995. "Women's Reactions to Miscarriage: The Role of Attributes, Coping Styles, and Knowledge," *Journal of Applied Social Psychology* 25:59–76.

Johnson, Mark. 1993. *Moral Imagination: Implications of Cognitive Science for Ethics*. Chicago: University of Chicago Press.

Johnston, Mark. 1988. "Self-Deception and the Nature of Mind." In McLaughlin and Rorty, eds.

Jones, Karen. 1996. "Trust as an Affective Attitude," *Ethics* 107:4–25.

Kass, Nancy, Jeremy Sugarman, Ruth Faden, and Monica Schoch-Spana. 1996. "Trust: The Fragile Foundation of Contemporary Biomedical Research," *Hastings Center Report* 26(5):25–29.

Kay, Margarita Artschwager. 1980. "Mexican, Mexican American, and Chicana Childbirth." In *Twice a Minority: Mexican American Women*. Ed. Margarita B. Melville. St. Louis: Mosby.

Kittay, Eva Feder. 1999. *Love's Labor: Essays on Women, Equality, and Dependency*. New York: Routledge.

Kornblith, Hilary. 1998. "What Is it Like to Be Me?" *Australasian Journal of Philosophy* 76(1):48–60.

Kurjak, Asim, ed. 1985. *The Fetus as a Patient*. Amsterdam: Elsevier Science.

Lasker, J. and L. Toedter. 1994. "Satisfaction with Hospital Care and Interventions after Pregnancy Loss," *Death Studies* 18:41–64.

Layne, Linda. 1990. "Motherhood Lost: Cultural Dimensions of Miscarrige and Stillbirth in America," *Women and Health* 16(¾):69–98.

Lazarus, Ellen. 1994. "What Do Women Want? Issues of Choice, Control, and Class in Pregnancy and Childbirth," *Medical Anthropology Quarterly* 8:25–46.

Leaney, Cindy and Michelle Silver (producers, directors). 1995. *Unsung Lullabies* (film). Vancouver, BC: No Time to Cry Productions.

Lehrer, Keith. 1997. *Self-Trust: A Study of Reason, Knowledge, and Autonomy*. New York: Oxford University Press.

Lepine, Diane. 1990. "Ending the Cycle of Violence: Overcoming Guilt in Incest Survivors." In *Healing Voices: Feminist Approaches to Therapy with Women*. Eds. Toni Ann Laidlaw, Cheryl Malmo, and associates. San Francisco: Jossey-Bass.

Lidz, Charles, Paul Appelbaum, and Alan Meisel. 1988. "Two Models of Implementing Informed Consent," *Archives of Internal Medicine* 1481(June): 1385–1389.

Lugones, Maria. 1987. "Playfulness, 'World'-Travelling, and Loving Perception," *Hypatia* 2(2):3–19.

Luhmann, Niklas. 1998. "Familiarity, Confidence, Trust: Problems and Alternatives." In *Trust: Making and Breaking Cooperative Relations*. Ed. Diego Gambetta. New York: Basil Blackwell.

Mackenzie, Catriona. 1992. "Abortion and Embodiment," *Australian Journal of Philosophy* 70(2): 136–155.

———. 2000. "Imaging Oneself Otherwise." In Mackenzie and Stoljar, eds.

Mackenzie, Catriona and Natalie Stoljar, eds. 2000. *Relational Autonomy: Feminist Perspectives on Autonomy, Agency, and the Social Self*. New York: Oxford University Press.

Madden, Margaret. 1994. "The Variety of Emotional Reactions to Miscarriage," *Women and Health* 21(2/3): 85–104.

Mattingly, Susan. 1992. "The Maternal-Fetal Dyad: Exploring the Two-Patient Obstetric Model," *Hastings Center Report* 22(1): 13–18.

May, Larry, Marilyn Friedman, and Andy Clark, eds. 1996. *Mind and Morals: Essays on Ethics and Cognitive Science*. Cambridge: MIT Press.

McFall, Lynne. 1987. "Integrity," *Ethics* 98:5–20.

McLaughlin, Brian and Amelie Oksenberg Rorty, eds. 1988. *Perspectives on Self-Deception*. Berkeley: University of California Press.

McLeod, Carolyn. 1998. "Women's Autonomy and the 'G' Case," *Canadian Bioethics Society Newsletter* 3(2):6.

———. 2000. "Our Attitude Towards the Motivation of Those We Trust," *Southern Journal of Philosophy* 38(3): 465–479.

——— and Lee Harris. n.d. "Administering Infertility Treatments: A Feminist Narrative of Objectification." Unpublished Manuscript.

——— and Susan Sherwin. 2000. "Relational Autonomy, Self-Trust, and Health Care for Patients Who are Oppressed." In MacKenzie and Stoljar, eds.

Mennuti, Michael. 1996. "A 35-Year-Old Pregnant Woman Considering Maternal Serum Screening and Amniocentesis," *Journal of the American Medical Association* 275(18): 1440–1446.

Mentor, Steven. 1998. "Witches, Nurses, Midwives, and Cyborgs: IVF, ART, and Complex Agency in the World of Technobirth." In Davis-Floyd and Dumit, eds.

Meyers, Diana T. 1987. "The Socialized Individual and Individual Autonomy: An Intersection between Philosophy and Psychology." In *Women and Moral Theory*. Eds. Eva Feder Kittay and Diana T. Meyers. Totowa NJ: Rowman & Littlefield.

———. 1989. *Self, Society, and Personal Choice*. New York: Columbia University Press.

————. 1994. *Subjection and Subjectivity: Psychoanalytic Feminism and Moral Philosophy*. New York: Routledge.

————, ed. 1997. *Feminists Rethink the Self*. Boulder: Westview Press.

————. 2000. "Intersectional Identity and the Authentic Self?: Opposites Attract!" In Mackenzie and Stoljar, eds.

Miller, Susan. 1985. *The Shame Experience*. Hillsdale, NJ: Analytic Press.

Mitchell, Lisa and Eugenia Georges. 1998. "Baby's First Picture: The Cyborg Fetus of Ultrasound Imaging." In Davis-Floyd and Dumit, eds.

Morgan, Kathryn Pauly. 1989. "Of *Woman* Born? How Old-fashioned!— New Reproductive Technologies and Women's Oppression." In Overall, ed.

Murphy, Julien S. 1999. "Should Lesbians Count as Infertile Couples? Antilesbian Discrimination in Assisted Reproduction." In Donchin and Purdy, eds.

Nagel, Thomas. 1986. *The View from Nowhere*. New York: Oxford University Press.

Nedelsky, Jennifer. 1989. "Reconceiving Autonomy: Sources, Thoughts, and Possibilities," *Yale Journal of Law and Feminism* 1(1): 7–36.

Neugebauer, R, J. Kline, P. O'Connor, P. Shrout, J. Johnson, A. Skodol, J. Wicks, and M. Susser. 1992. "Determinants of Depressive Symptoms in the Early Weeks after Miscarriage," *American Journal of Public Health* 82(10): 1332–1339.

Nsiah-Jefferson, Laurie. 1994. "Reproductive Genetic Services for Low-Income Women and Women of Color: Access and Sociocultural Issues." In Rothenberg and Thomson, eds.

Overall, Christine, ed. 1987. *Ethics and Human Reproduction*. Boston: Allen & Unwin.

————. 1993. *Human Reproduction: Principles, Practices, Policies*. Toronto: Oxford University Press.

Pateman, Carole. 1988. *The Sexual Contract*. Stanford: Stanford University Press.

Pellegrino, Edmund. 1991. "Trust and Distrust in Professional Ethics." In Pellegrino, Veatch, and Langan eds.

Pellegrino, Edmund, Robert Veatch, and John Langan, eds. 1991. *Ethics, Trust, and the Professions*. Washington: Georgetown University Press.

Petchesky, Rosalind Pollack. 1987. "Foetal Images: The Power of Visual Culture in the Politics of Reproduction." In *Reproductive Technologies: Gender, Motherhood, and Medicine,* Ed. Michelle Stanworth. Cambridge: Polity Press.

Pollock, John. 1986. *Contemporary Theories of Knowledge*. Totowa, NJ: Rowman & Littlefield.

Puddifoot, J.E. and M.P. Johnson. 1997. "The Legitimacy of Grieving: The Partner's Experience of Miscarriage," *Social Science and Medicine* 45(6): 837–845.

Rajan, Lynda and Ann Oakley. 1993. "No Pills for Heartache: The Importance of Social Support for Women Who Suffer Pregnancy Loss," *Journal of Reproductive and Infant Psychology* 11: 75–87.

Rapp, Rayna. 1993. "Amniocentesis in Sociocultural Perspective," *Journal of Genetic Counseling* 2: 183–195.

———. 1997. "Constructing Amniocentesis: Maternal and Medical Discourses." In *Situated Lives: Gender and Culture in Everyday Life.* Eds. L. Lamphere, H. Ragone, and P. Zarella. New York: Routledge.

———. 1998. "Refusing Prenatal Diagnosis: The Uneven Meanings of Bioscience in a Multicultural World." In Davis-Floyd and Dumit, eds.

Roberts, Cathy. 1989. *Women and Rape.* New York: New York University Press.

Roberts, Dorothy. 1997. *Killing the Black Body: Race, Reproduction, and the Meaning of Liberty.* New York: Pantheon Books.

Robertson, John. 1994. *Children of Choice: Freedom and the New Reproductive Technologies.* Princeton: Princeton University Press.

Robinson, Bambi. 1997. "Birds Do It. Bees Do It. So Why Not Single Women and Lesbians?" *Bioethics* 11(3–4): 217–227.

Rorty, Amelie Oksenberg. 1980. "Explaining Emotions." In *Explaining Emotions.* Ed. Amelie O. Rorty. Berkeley: University of California Press.

———. 1994. "User-Friendly Self-Deception," *Philosophy* 69: 211–228.

———. 1998. "The Deceptive Self: Liars, Layers, and Lairs." In McLaughlin and Rorty, eds.

Rossing, M. A., J. R. Daling, N.S. Weiss, D.E. Moore, and S.G. Self. 1994. "Ovarian tumor in a cohort of infertile women," *New England Journal of Medicine* 331(12): 771–776.

Rothenberg, Karen and Elizabeth Thomson, eds. 1994. *Women and Prenatal Testing: Facing the Challenges of Genetic Technology.* Columbus: Ohio State University Press.

Rothman, Barbara Katz. 1986. *The Tentative Pregnancy: Prenatal Diagnosis and the Future of Motherhood.* New York: Viking.

———. 1989. *Recreating Motherhood: Ideology and Technology in a Patriarchal Society.* New York: Norton.

Royal Commission on New Reproductive Technologies. 1993. *Proceed with Care: Final Report of the Royal Commission.* Vol. 1. Ottawa: Minister of Government Services, Canada.

Ruddick, William. 1988. "Social Self-Deceptions." In McLaughlin and Rorty, eds.

Russell, Dianne. 1986. *The Secret Trauma.* New York: Basic Books.

Scheman, Naomi. 1983. "Individualism and the Objects of Psychology." In *Discovering Reality: Feminist Perspectives on Epistemology, Metaphysics, Methodology, and Philosophy of Science.* Eds. Sandra Harding and Merrill B. Hintikka. Boston: Reidel.

————. 1993. "Though this Be Method, Yet There Is Madness in It: Paranoia and Liberal Epistemology." In *Engenderings: Constructions of Knowledge, Authority, and Privilege.* Ed. Naomi Scheman. New York: Routledge.

————. 2001. "Epistemology Resuscitated: Objectivity as Trustworthiness." In *Engendering Rationalities.* Eds. Nancy Tuana and Sandra Morgen. Albany, NY: SUNY Press.

Shanner, Laura. 1996. "Bioethics through the Back Door: Phenomenology, Narratives, and Insights into Infertility." In *Philosophical Perspectives on Bioethics.* Eds. L. W. Sumner and Joseph Boyle. Toronto: University of Toronto Press.

Sherwin, Susan. 1998. "A Relational Approach to Autonomy in Health Care." In *The Feminist Health Care Ethics Research Network.*

Sjogren, B. and N. Uddenberg. 1988. "Decision-making During the Prenatal Diagnostic Procedure: A Questionnaire and Interview Study of 211 Women Participating in Prenatal Diagnosis," *Prenatal Diagnosis* 8: 263–273.

Smith, Eva Marie. 1993. "Race or Racism? Addiction in the United States," *Annals of Epidemiology* 3(2): 165–170.

Smith, Janet Farrell. 1996. "Communicative Ethics in Medicine: The Physician-Patient Relationship." In *Feminism and Bioethics: Beyond Reproduction.* Ed. Susan M. Wolf. New York: Oxford University Press.

Steele, Claude, 1995. "Stereotype Threat and the Intellectual Test Performance of African Americans," *Journal of Personality and Social Psychology* 69(5): 797–811.

————. 1997. "A Threat in the Air: How Stereotypes Shape Intellectual Identity and Performance," *American Psychologist* 52(6): 613–629.

Stewart, D. and A. Cecutti. 1993. "Physical Abuse in Pregnancy," *Canadian Medical Association Journal* 149(9): 1257–1263.

Stoljar, Natalie. 1996. "Procedural Autonomy and the Requirement of Self-Knowledge." Unpublished manuscript.

————. 2000. "Autonomy and the Feminist Intuition." In Mackenzie and Stoljart, eds.

Taylor, Charles. 1985. "Atomism." In *Philosophy and the Human Sciences: Philosophical Papers* 2. Cambridge: Cambridge University Press.

The Feminist Health Care Ethics Research Network. 1998. *The Politics of Women's Health: Exploring Agency and Autonomy.* Philadelphia: Temple University Press.

Thomson, Judith Jarvis. 1971. "A Defense of Abortion," *Philosophy and Public Affairs* 1: 47–66.

Walker, Margaret Urban. 1998. *Moral Understandings: A Feminist Study in Ethics.* New York: Routledge.

Warren, Mary Anne. 1975. "On the Moral and Legal Status of Abortion." In *Today's Moral Problems.* Ed. R. Wasserstrom. London: Macmillan.

Webb, Mark Owen. 1992. "The Epistemology of Trust and the Politics of Suspicion," *Pacific Philosophical Quarterly* 73:390–400.

Wertz, D.C., J.M. Rosenfield, S.R. Janes, and R.W. Erbe. 1991. "Attitudes Toward Abortion among Parents of Children with Cystic Fibrosis," *American Journal of Public Health* 81(8): 922–996.

Whitbeck, Caroline. 1995. "Trust." *The Encyclopedia of Bioethics,* 2nd ed. New York: Macmillan.

Wilkerson, Abby. 1998. " 'Her Body Her Own Worst Enemy': The Medicalization of Violence Against Women." In *Violence Against Women: Philosophical Perspectives.* Eds. Stanley French, Wanda Teays, and Laura Purdy. Ithaca: Cornell University Press.

Williams, Bernard. 1981. "Persons, Character, and Morality" and "Moral Luc." In *Moral Luck: Philosophical Papers 1973–1980.* New York: Cambridge University Press.

Williams, Linda. 1989. "No Relief Until the End: The Physical and Emotional Costs of in Vitro Fertilization." In Overall, ed.

Wolf, Susan. 1989. "Sanity and the Metaphysics of Responsibility." In Christman, ed.

Young, Iris Marion. 1990. *Justice and the Politics of Difference.* Princeton, NJ: Princeton University Press.

Young, Robert. 1989. "Autonomy and the 'Inner Self.'" In Christman, ed.

Zaner, Richard. 1991. "The Phenomenon of Trust and the Patient-Physician Relationship." In Pellegrino, Veatch, and Langar, eds.

Index

Roberts, Cathy, 69
Roberts, Dorothy, 2, 71, 117
Robertson, John, 114
Rorty, Amelie O., 81, 94
Rothman, Barbara K., 145
Royal Commission, 118, 119
Russell, Dianne, 69

Scheman, Naomi, 70, 75
Second-order reflection, 107, 109,
  168n.11
Second trimester abortion, 145–146
Self
  fragmentation of, 154
  relation to the body, 3, 49–50, 56, 65
  sociopolitical (feminist), 105
Self-betrayal, 67–68
Self-confidence, 51–52
Self-deception, 68, 94–94
Self-direction, 105, 107–108,
  126–127
Self-distrust, 45, 139, 155. *See also*
  Self-trust
  authenticity and, 119–121
  as broken self-trust, 39–42
  choice and, 114–118, 131
  justified, 95–97, 163–164,
  172–173n.1
  vulnerability of, 70–71
Self-distrust (case illustrations)
  Eve (obstetrics), 95–98, 99, 100
  Lara (prenatal screening), 140–143,
  144, 145, 149, 164
Self-knowledge
  as a condition of autonomy,
  126–129, 131, 140
  social feedback and, 73–77, 93–95,
  96
Self-reliance, 51, 169n.16
Self-respect/self-worth, 52, 69, 109,
  113, 162, 163
Self-trust. *See also* Patient self-trust;
  Self-distrust; Trust
  autonomy and, 9, 46, 60, 103–106,
  129–131, 163

defined and characterized, 35, 46,
  49–52, 88
epistemic competence and, 40, 41–42
excessive or unjustified, 161–163
future expectations and, 48–49
justified, 8–9, 104, 109, 126–130
moral component of, 40–41, 47,
  56–57, 104
relational aspect of, 6–7, 9, 12–15,
  36–42, 52–56
trauma or abuse affecting, 69–70
Sex differences, 169n.3
Sexism. *See also* Feminist perspective;
  Oppressive social environments
  sexist attitudes in medical
  environment, 4, 9, 39–40
  sexist norms, 79, 84, 89–90, 96, 99
  sexist paradigm scenarios, 99
Shanner, Laura, 116, 118
Sherwin. Susan, 101, 119
  on social influences on autonomy, 9,
  110, 111, 112, 113
Sickle-cell screening, 116
Smith, Janet F., 135
Smoking cessation during pregnancy,
  161–162
Social class or classism. *See also*
  Oppressive social relations
  case illustration (Melissa), 150–153
Social epistemology, defined, 93
Social feedback, 93–95, 96
  reliability of, 97, 98–99
Social pathology, 113
Social reliabilism, 8, 94–95, 97–99
Social workers, 139, 144
Steele, Claude, 153
Stereotypes. *See also* Objectification
  affecting physician-patient
  relationship, 134, 139, 150–152
  affecting self-trust or distrust, 71,
  75–76
  context or "world" dependent
  responses to, 151–152
  oppressive, 87, 110, 114, 128–129,
  170n.6